Essential Pathology for Dental Students

Essential Pathology for Dental Students

William Lawler

MD MRCPath
Senior Lecturer in Pathology, University of Manchester

Ali Ahmed

MD
Senior Lecturer in Pathology, University of Manchester

William J Hume

PhD BDS FDSRCPS MRCPath
Professor of Dental Surgery, School of Dentistry, University
of Leeds. Formerly Senior Lecturer and Honorary Consultant
in Oral Pathology, University of Manchester

CHURCHILL LIVINGSTONE
EDINBURGH LONDON MELBOURNE AND NEW YORK 1987

CHURCHILL LIVINGSTONE
Medical Division of Longman Group UK Limited

Distributed in the United States of America by Churchill
Livingstone Inc., 1560 Broadway, New York, N.Y. 10036,
and by associated companies, branches and representatives
throughout the world.

First published 1987

ISBN 0-443-02910-5

British Library Cataloguing in Publication Data
Lawler, William
    Essential pathology for dental students.
    — (Churchill Livingstone dental series).
    1. Pathology
    I. Title   II. Ahmed, Ali   III. Hume,
William J.
    616.07′0246176   RB111

    ISBN 0-443-02910-5

Library of Congress Cataloging in Publication Data
Lawler, William
    Essential pathology for dental students.
    (Dental series)
    Includes index.
    1. Pathology.   2. Dental students.   I. Ahmed, Ali.
II. Hume, William J.   III. Title.   IV. Series:
Churchill Livingstone dental series.   [DNLM:
1. Pathology.   QZ 4 L418e]
RB112.L38   1987   616.07′0246176   87-10323
ISBN 0-443-02910-5 (pbk.)

Produced by Longman Singapore Publishers (Pte) Ltd.
Printed in Singapore.

Preface

This book is intended to provide the essentials of pathology for dental students. Its contents are based on the dental pathology course in Manchester, and they comply with the recommendations of the Nuffield Foundation conference, held in October 1981, on the 'Medical Teaching of Dental Students'.

We are convinced that a good knowledge and understanding of pathology and pathological concepts form a sound basis for subsequent clinical practice. The book is designed in two parts: the first deals with the principles of general pathology, while the second covers appropriate selected aspects of systemic pathology.

Our teaching in Manchester reflects the importance of an oral pathologist's contribution to teaching pathology to dental students. Many dental students find it difficult to understand why they are taught so much pathology, and we therefore consider it very important to include and to emphasise specific dental examples to illustrate the relevance of the disease processes being discussed. Thus, this book contains many such examples; in some chapters they are appended at the end, whilst in others they are incorporated into the main body of the text.

In our experience, black and white illustrations are not particularly helpful to undergraduates, and we believe that pathology is best illustrated in colour (in lectures) and in mounted specimens (in practical classes); furthermore, suitable colour texts are now available for reference if required.

The depth of coverage between individual chapters varies considerably, and this reflects the relative importance which we attach to their contents. Thus, as immunopathological mechanisms become more important in understanding common dental diseases (e.g. gingivitis and periodontitis), a sound knowledge of the basic principles involved is essential. Similarly, we consider bone, mucocutaneous and haematological diseases to be particularly important. We have attempted to overcome our criticism of the usual teaching of radiation effects by including an elementary discussion of radiobiology. Nervous system diseases are often fragmented throughout the dental curriculum, and we felt it useful to provide an overview of this subject for the students' present and future use.

This book is not meant to be definitive and comprehensive. Our intention has been to try to write a concise, inexpensive, basic pathology text sufficient for any dental student's requirements; we hope that, when used in conjunction with lectures, tutorials and practical teaching, it will provide the pathological basis for all subsequent clinical subjects.

Contents

1 Introduction   1

2 Cell damage   4

3 Inflammation   7

4 Healing   12

5 Infections   15

6 Immunopathology   24

7 Miscellaneous tissue deposits   32

8 Circulatory disturbances   35

9 Disorders of cell growth and development   39

10 Neoplasia   42

11 Effects of radiation   48

12 Vascular diseases   52

13 Cardiac diseases   57

14 Respiratory diseases   62

15 Diseases of the mouth and salivary glands   69

16 Alimentary diseases   75

17 Hepatic, biliary and pancreatic diseases   82

18 Urinary tract diseases   91

19 Endocrine diseases   100

20 Haematological diseases   104

21 Diseases of the lymphoreticular system   113

22 Bone diseases   117

23 Joint, muscle and connective tissue diseases   123

24 Nervous system diseases   128

25 Mucocutaneous diseases   138

Index   144

1

Introduction

Pathology
Basic terminology in pathology
Causes of disease
Genetic diseases
Acquired diseases
Useful approach to pathology

PATHOLOGY

Pathology is the scientific study of disease, its causes and its effects; disease is any disturbance of normal body structure or function.

Pathological changes are neither constant nor static as there is always continual interaction between the causative agent or agents and the body's natural responses; nevertheless, fairly consistent patterns emerge, and these are the foundations of pathological practice.

As pathology constitutes study of diseases, it follows that pathological abnormalities form the basis for all clinical conditions. A good knowledge and understanding of pathology and pathological processes, therefore, provide an important background for sound and accurate clinical diagnosis, and pathology is always extremely relevant to all aspects of clinical practice.

Several branches of pathology exist. This book is concerned mainly with *anatomical pathology* as encountered in *surgical pathology* (the study of organs, tissues or biopsies removed by clinicians), *morbid anatomy* (post mortem examination—i.e. *autopsy* or *necropsy*) and *histopathology* (microscopical examination of tissues); features of other branches, including *haematology* (study of blood cells and their diseases), *biochemistry* (analyses of changes in biochemical constituents of body fluids, especially blood) and *microbiology* (study of microorganisms responsible for infectious diseases) are discussed where appropriate.

BASIC TERMINOLOGY IN PATHOLOGY

Throughout this book, several basic terms, applicable to most diseases and many pathological processes, are used repeatedly, and justify brief consideration and definition here.

Aetiology is the actual cause or causes of the disease.

Pathogenesis is the sequence of events in disease development from outset to termination, and includes any influencing factors; thus, it is the means whereby the aetiological agent brings about disease. Although not synonymous, aetiology and pathogenesis are usually considered together.

Predisposing factors are pre-existing pathological or physiological states which increase the likelihood of developing the disease.

Natural history is the 'normal' course of any disease, unmodified and unaffected by treatment, from beginning to end.

Symptoms are abnormalities or subjective complaints noticed by the patient.

Physical signs are abnormalities found or elicited on clinical examination. Some diseases may be well established or even fairly advanced before symptoms and/or physical signs appear.

Lesions are the pathological structural abnormalities. They may be *macroscopical* (i.e. visible on naked eye examination) or *microscopical* (i.e. detectable only by appropriate microscopy).

Diagnosis is an opinion, based on all available evidence, of the disease process or processes present. Anyone can attempt to make a diagnosis; often, it is relatively easy, but sometimes considerable experience and numerous different investi-

1

gational techniques are necessary; rarely, only a list of possible diseases can be provided (i.e. *differential diagnoses*), with further tests required before an accurate *definitive diagnosis* can be made.

Prognosis is a prediction of the likely outcome of any disease, and is obviously influenced by treatment given.

Morbidity reflects ill-health, incapacity or sickness associated with non-fatal disease.

Mortality relates to deaths from disease.

CAUSES OF DISEASE

These are numerous and diverse, and many diseases have more than one cause. When cause or causes are unknown, adequate prevention is impossible.

All known causes are either *genetic* or *acquired*; both may be *congenital* (i.e. develop during intra-uterine life and present at birth) or may develop some time after birth (often many years).

Genetic diseases

These reflect underlying abnormalities of DNA structure or errors in its transcription. Most are due to single abnormal genes, which may be inherited from one or both parents or which may arise spontaneously by *mutation*. The inheritance pattern of these abnormal genes may be relatively simple (as a *dominant* from one parent; as a *recessive* from both parents, one or both of whom may be free from the disease; as an *X-linked* disease, which an affected male receives on the X chromosome from an unaffected, 'carrier' mother) or complex, where the disease runs in families but where no straightforward mode of inheritance can be determined (i.e. a *familial tendency*). A few show gross chromosomal defects (e.g. additional chromosomes, deletion of chromosome components or translocation of chromosomal fragments); these are usually associated with multiple, severe congenital abnormalities, which are often rapidly fatal.

Acquired diseases

Many causes exist, and often there is a complex interrelationship between two or more of these factors in any one disease process; some important factors are discussed briefly below and in more detail in later sections and chapters.

Infections. These are due to pathogenic micro-organisms, and are widespread, common and important causes of disease (Chapter 5).

Physical agents. These produce disease by energy transfer, and include mechanical injury (trauma), burns, heat and cold (Chapter 2), electricity and radiation (Chapter 11).

Chemicals. Numerous chemicals, both organic and inorganic, are widely available in industry, agriculture and the home. A few are *toxic* and produce disease ranging from reversible mild inflammation at the entry site to irreversible localised or generalised cell death; their long term accumulation within the body may, in some instances, cause neoplasia (Chapter 10). *Drugs*, chemicals used for treatment, may cause additional disease, particularly if abnormally handled by the body or taken in excessive quantities.

Nutritional deficiencies. These usually reflect inadequate dietary intake, and include proteins, vitamins, minerals, salts and fat. Absolute deficiencies (*starvation* or *malnutrition*) are common in many countries; in more affluent areas, nutritional deficiencies often reflect alimentary tract diseases (*malabsorption*—Chapter 16), and excessive intake (*obesity*) causes other problems.

Immunological disturbances. These produce hypersensitivity reactions and auto-immune diseases (Chapter 6).

Mechanical factors. Factors causing luminal obstruction within body systems (e.g. urinary, alimentary and respiratory tracts) will produce disease elsewhere in the system affected.

Metabolic abnormalities. These reflect local or general physiological disturbances, and include nutritional deficiency states (see above), miscellaneous tissue deposits (Chapter 7) and endocrine dysfunctions (Chapter 19).

Circulatory disturbances. Disturbances due to vascular and cardiac diseases are discussed in Chapter 8.

Age. Degenerative changes due simply to ageing are fairly common and contribute to many diseases in elderly patients.

Neoplasms. These are probably due to one or more of the above factors, and cause associated local and sometimes widespread tissue damage and disease (Chapter 10).

Psychosomatic factors. These include prolonged stress, fear, anxiety and frustration, and may cause or contribute to several diseases, particularly in more affluent countries, although the mechanisms whereby they act are largely unknown.

Iatrogenic diseases. These are directly attributable to medical or surgical treatment, and may be predictable or unexpected (i.e. idiosyncratic reactions).

Idiopathic diseases. Although knowledge of factors causing disease has expanded remarkably over the last 50 years, there are still many diseases where cause or causes remain unknown—that is, they are *idiopathic*. Sometimes, idiopathic diseases are designated *primary*, in contrast to *secondary diseases*, which have recognised causes.

USEFUL APPROACH TO PATHOLOGY

It is always very useful (and in examinations, important) to have a logical and systematic approach to pathological conditions and diseases, and it is well worth while developing such an approach at the outset. Below is the outline of a series of questions worth applying to any pathological entity.

Definition. A clear, concise and accurate definition of the appropriate condition is an essential starting point.

Incidence. How common is it? A knowledge of the approximate incidence of different conditions enables anyone to put them into perspective and into order of frequency. The old adage that common things are common will always be applicable to pathology, and it is important to begin by discussing the most likely possibilities.

Aetiology. What is the cause? Is more than one cause known? Is it idiopathic? Are any predisposing factors recognised?

Pathogenesis. What is the natural sequence of events in its evolution? Are any influencing factors known?

Age. When does it usually develop—infancy, childhood, old age, etc.? Can it appear at any age?

Sex. Is it obviously more common in males or females, or is the sex incidence approximately equal?

Geographical distribution. Is it more common in particular areas or countries? Is this related to affluence, poverty, climatic conditions or certain socio-economic groups?

Lesions. What does it look like macroscopically? What are the microscopic appearances? Are these features specific for the disease concerned? What is required for a definitive clinical or pathological diagnosis? Is a differential diagnosis appropriate?

Clinical features. What are the usual presenting symptoms? What physical signs are found? How specific are these features? Are they diagnostic? Are any other investigations (radiology, biochemistry, microbiology, etc.) diagnostic?

Spread. Does it spread locally? Does distant spread occur? How does it spread? What effects does spread produce?

Treatment. Does any treatment exist? How specific and how effective is treatment? Are there significant side effects?

Prognosis. What is the natural history? What is the likely outcome? What factors influence prognosis? What complications may develop? Does it predispose to any other disease?

2

Cell damage

Introduction
General features
Degenerations
Infiltrations
Necrosis

Specific injuries
Burns
Heat
Cold
Radiation

INTRODUCTION

Cell damage may result from various causes and may be manifest structurally in several ways. Early or mild injury produces either an excessive accumulation of normal metabolites (*degeneration*) or an accumulation of abnormal products (*infiltration*); these changes indicate functional derangement but are reversible if the initiating factors are removed. If severe or prolonged, irreversible cell death results.

Causes of cell damage include hypoxia (usually due to impairment of blood supply), bacterial or viral infections, immunological injury, toxins, enzyme deficiencies, chemical poisons and physical agents (cold, heat, radiation and mechanical trauma).

GENERAL FEATURES

Degenerations

These are due to sublethal damage and disruption within the various cellular components—the cell membrane is abnormally permeable, the endoplasmic reticulum and mitochondria are swollen and show loss of granules, polyribosomes are disaggregated and lysosomes are ruptured. In addition, there may be alteration in intracytoplasmic organelles in an attempt to eradicate or neutralise the causative agent.

Degenerations are usually given purely descriptive names, depending on cytoplasmic appearances.

Cloudy swelling is the earliest change, and indicates swollen, hazy, granular cytoplasm.

Hydropic degeneration implies excess intracytoplasmic fluid, and is seen as one or more clear vacuoles.

Hyaline degeneration represents advanced cellular damage, and in practice is usually irreversible. Here, the cytoplasm is uniformly eosinophilic (i.e. it appears pink in routine haematoxylin- and eosin-stained histological preparations) and rather 'glassy'.

Infiltrations

Of these, excess fat accumulation (*fatty change*) is the most important, and is seen as intracytoplasmic lipid droplets. *Inborn errors of metabolism*, due to specific enzyme deficiencies, may cause infiltration by particular substances (e.g. glucocerebrosides in Gaucher's disease and various forms of glycogen in the glycogen storage diseases).

Necrosis

Necrosis indicates irreversible cell death. The cytoplasmic changes are often those of degeneration (see above), but, in addition, co-existing, characteristic nuclear changes are seen. Initially, the nucleus shrinks and shows clumping and increased density of its chromatin (*pyknosis*). The nuclear membrane then ruptures, with chromatin fragmentation (*karyorrhexis*). Finally, nuclear material is digested and disappears (*karyolysis*). Once cell death has occurred, there is severe structural disorganisation and ultimate disappearance of cytoplasmic organelles due to digestion by intracellular lytic enzymes (*autolysis*).

Several types of necrosis are described:

Coagulative necrosis. This is the commonest, and shows preservation of cellular outlines in the necrotic tissue.

Apoptosis. This is a form of individual cell death subtly different from coagulative necrosis (Table 2.1). Following nuclear condensation, the cell 'bursts' into several small membrane-bound fragments of nuclear and/or cytoplasmic material (apoptotic bodies), which are then either phagocytosed and digested by adjacent tissue cells or macrophages, or extruded on to luminal surfaces. Although it is usually seen in abnormal circumstances (e.g. malignant tumours, adrenal gland atrophy, irradiated tissues and following steroid or cytotoxic drug administration), it also occurs in normal tissues (e.g. gastrointestinal epithelium), and provides a means of deleting cells during intra-uterine development.

Caseous necrosis. Characteristic of tuberculosis, this is associated with loss of cell outlines.

Colliquative necrosis. This indicates softening and liquefaction of dead cells, and is found in the central nervous system.

Fat necrosis. This follows irreversible damage to fat cells, and is usually due either to traumatic rupture or to local release of lipase enzymes (as in acute pancreatitis—Chapter 17).

Suppurative necrosis. Suppurative necrosis (i.e. with pus formation) is encountered with acute inflammation due to pyogenic bacteria capable of secreting local tissue-destroying enzymes (Chapter 3).

Fibrinoid 'necrosis'. This is associated with the accumulation of strongly eosinophilic, fibrin-like material (hence its name). It was originally thought to represent collagen necrosis, but is now believed to include local fibrin formation following vascular leakage of fibrinogen and other proteins from the plasma (a process sometimes designated *plasmatic vasculosis*); true necrosis is not a feature. It is seen in some hypersensitivity reactions (Chapter 6) and malignant hypertension (Chapter 12).

Gangrene. Gangrene is extensive necrosis (e.g. of limbs or segments of bowel).

Wet gangrene indicates infection and digestion of necrotic tissue by saprophytic bacteria (i.e. bacteria unable to reproduce in living tissues)—a process known as *putrefaction*. These organisms break down cellular constituents to produce, amongst other substances, foul-smelling gases. The tissue is markedly swollen and almost black in colour.

Dry gangrene is a more gradual process, unassociated with saprophytic infection and putrefaction, which is sometimes designated *mummification*; the tissue slowly shrinks and dries.

Gas gangrene is a specific infection caused by the Clostridia group of anaerobic, spore-bearing bacteria, usually *Clostridium welchii*. The spores contaminate penetrating wounds, and if the environment is favourable, they proliferate and produce powerful exotoxins and proteolytic enzymes which destroy adjacent tissues. Without early and adequate local treatment, organism dissemination occurs; this, together with severe toxaemia, soon proves fatal.

Infarction. *Infarction* is ischaemic necrosis due to impaired blood supply; it is considered with circulatory disturbances in Chapter 8.

SPECIFIC INJURIES

Burns

Burns result from heat applied to the body, and may be caused by dry heat (as in fire), hot liquids and steam (scalds), electricity, chemicals and irradiation. Two major degrees exist—*partial thickness* (involving only superficial epidermal layers) and *full thickness* (extending through epidermis into deeper structures, with or without involvement of such tissues as muscle and bone). Partial thickness burns heal by regeneration without permanent damage; full thickness burns

Table 2.1 Differences between coagulative necrosis and apoptosis

Coagulative necrosis	Apoptosis
1. Affects groups of cells	1. Affects single cells
2. Followed by inflammation	2. Not followed by inflammation
3. Cells remain intact with a 'ghosted appearance'	3. Cells fragment into membrane-bound apoptotic bodies
4. Enzyme activity lost	4. Enzyme activity retained

initiate inflammation (Chapter 3) and heal by secondary intention with excess scar tissue formation (Chapter 4). The extent and degree of burning reflect duration and severity of the causative agent. With extensive full thickness burns, there is marked associated plasma loss producing electrolyte disturbances, haemoconcentration and hypovolaemic shock (Chapter 8); secondary bacterial infection is frequent. Prognosis is related directly to the surface area involved, but is also adversely influenced by increasing age, inadequate treatment (particularly in fluid replacement) and poor general physical health.

Heat

Localised, more intense heat produces burning; generalised, less intense heat causes heat stroke or heat exhaustion.

Heat stroke (*'sunstroke'*) occurs in very humid, tropical areas when the body's normal heat-regulating mechanisms fail because sweat evaporation is inadequate; hyperpyrexia results, with associated generalised cell damage and cell death.

Heat exhaustion occurs in a confined environment during prolonged, heavy physical exercise, and is due to excessive sweating with chloride depletion; characteristically, muscular cramps (*'stoker's cramps'*), giddiness and vomiting develop, and there may be hypovolaemic shock.

Cold

Cold may damage cells locally (to produce frost-bite or 'trench-foot') or generally (hypothermia); cryosurgery represents deliberate local tissue destruction by cold.

Frostbite. This is exposure to freezing temperatures. Ice crystals form within cells and tissues, and intravascular thrombosis develops; the result is local ischaemia, infarction and gangrene.

Trench-foot. 'Trench-foot' or 'Immersion-foot' results from prolonged exposure to low, non-freezing temperatures. There is local supression of vital cellular metabolic processes with cell damage or death; in addition, vascular damage occurs, with oedema formation and, in severe cases, thrombosis with ischaemia and infarction.

Cryosurgery. This is tissue destruction by a freezing probe. An ice-ball forms at the tip of the probe, and with prolonged application extends deeper into the tissue. The freezing and subsequent thawing of cells causes mechanical disruption and internal electrolyte imbalance, resulting in cell death. Advantages of cryosurgery include a reduction in postoperative scarring and the use in surgically difficult sites, for example the floor of the mouth. It is particularly suitable for superficial abnormalities, such as haemangiomas and leukoplakias, but can also be used in conjunction with conventional surgery, for example to kill residual tumour cells within bone.

Hypothermia. With generalised exposure to low temperatures, the initial reaction is marked peripheral vasoconstriction. Continued hypothermia produces loss of vasomotor tone, with vasodilatation, hyperaemia, cooling of peripheral blood and consequent circulatory failure; these cause depression of vital cerebral centres which, if prolonged, is irreversible and fatal.

Radiation

Cell damage following irradiation is considered separately in Chapter 11.

3

Inflammation

Introduction
Acute inflammation
Introduction
Causes
Macroscopic features
Microscopic events
Leucocytes involved

Acute inflammatory exudate
Mediators
Spread
Results
Chronic inflammation
Introduction
Causes

Cells involved
Granulomatous inflammation
Results
Dental aspects
Pulpitis
Periapical bone inflammation

INTRODUCTION

The inflammatory response is one of the most important natural defence mechanisms of the body, and is, simply, the body's response to tissue injury. It is initiated by numerous agents or stimuli and occurs in any part of the body, but its basic character is always the same, whatever the cause and whatever the site. The suffix *-itis* indicates inflammation whilst the prefix represents the organ or tissue involved—for example appendicitis and meningitis.

Traditionally, inflammation is divided into acute and chronic, but, in practice, these may overlap and both may appear together. 'Subacute inflammation' has no pathological meaning, although clinicians sometimes use the term when clinical signs and symptoms midway between acute and chronic inflammation are present.

ACUTE INFLAMMATION

Introduction

These are the initial or early changes, occurring over hours or days, and represent the body's attempt to destroy or neutralise the causative agent.

Causes

Common causes are listed in Table 3.1; the commonest is undoubtedly bacterial infection. Several are discussed in detail elsewhere—infections (Chapter 5), radiation (Chapter 11), extremes

Table 3.1 Causes of acute inflammation

Organisms—Bacteria
　　　　　—Viruses
　　　　　—Parasites
Mechanical trauma—Cutting
　　　　　　　　—Crushing
Chemicals—Inorganic—Strong acids
　　　　　　　　　　—Strong alkalis
　　　　—Organic
　　　　—Extravasated body fluids (e.g. bile and urine)
Radiation—Ionising
　　　　—Ultraviolet
Extremes of temperature—Cold
　　　　　　　　　　—Heat
Deprivation of blood supply—Infarction
Immunological reactions—Immune complexes

of temperature (Chapter 2), immunological reactions (Chapter 6) and infarction (Chapter 8).

Macroscopic features

These constitute the cardinal signs attributed to Celsus and comprise *tumor* (swelling), *rubor* (redness), *calor* (excess local heat) and *dolor* (pain). In addition, *functio laesa* (loss of function) may also develop.

Microscopic events

These relate to dynamic changes in blood vessels, blood flow and leucocyte activity. They usually occur sequentially and may be listed.

1. *Transient arteriolar constriction*, probably due to a local neurogenic reflex, may develop, but lasts only for a few minutes. It is rapidly followed by

2. *Prolonged arteriolar dilatation.* There is, therefore,

3. *Increased local blood flow (hyperaemia)* and local capillary bed dilatation.

4. *Increased capillary permeability* is due to two main factors. Firstly, arteriolar dilatation raises the capillary hydrostatic pressure, promoting greater outflow of water and solutes into the interstitial fluid (Starling's hypothesis). Secondly, capillary and venular endothelial permeability is increased, allowing larger molecules, especially albumin, to enter interstitial tissues. These molecules alter local osmotic pressures and attract more water into the tissues. This accumulation of interstitial fluid ('inflammatory oedema') derived from the circulation produces

5. *Slowing of capillary blood flow* and intravascular haemoconcentration. The increased plasma protein concentration produces increased blood viscosity. This is followed by

6. *Loss of normal axial blood flow.* Normally, blood cells flow in the centre of the capillaries, with the relatively cell free plasma in contact with the endothelium. In acute inflammation, circulating white cells, initially neutrophil polymorphs and later monocytes (see below), move outwards to produce

7. *Margination of leucocytes (Pavementing of endothelium)* and central

8. *'Sludging' of red cells*, forming rouleaux.

9. *Adhesion of leucocytes* to capillary endothelial cells then occurs, followed by active

10. *Emigration* by amoeboid movement, into perivascular tissues through gaps between endothelial cells. Once outside, they migrate by

11. *Chemotaxis*, a process whereby cells are attracted towards higher concentrations of certain chemical substances (*chemotaxins*). This active movement produces

12. *Accumulation* of numerous leucocytes at the appropriate site. This accumulation, so easily seen and recognised microscopically, is the main criterion for the histopathological diagnosis of acute inflammation.

13. *Phagocytosis* is the main function of these leucocytes; this is the ingestion, digestion and disposal of unwanted foreign particulate matter, especially bacteria and damaged host cells.

Leucocytes involved

Only two types are important. Initially, the vast majority are *neutrophil polymorphs*; they are highly motile, contain many lysosomes for digesting bacteria and effete cells, and are relatively short lived. Later, *macrophages* (derived from circulating monocytes) predominate; they are less motile, contain fewer lysosomes and remove debris, including dead polymorphs, bacteria and fibrin.

Acute inflammatory exudate

Constituents. The constituents of the acute inflammatory exudate are fluid, proteins and cells. The *fluid* is in constant exchange with the plasma; it may contain drugs (including antibiotics), and dilutes local irritant substances and toxins. The *proteins* include albumin, globulins (some of which may effect humoral-mediated immunity—Chapter 6) and fibrinogen. Fibrin (polymerised fibrinogen) helps to prevent bacterial invasion, unites severed tissues and promotes phagocytosis. The *cells*, mainly polymorphs and macrophages, are described above; with considerable local vascular damage, red cells may also accumulate in the tissues.

Types of acute inflammatory exudate. Several are described, including *serous* (mainly fluid), *fibrinous* (mainly fibrin and often seen on serosal surfaces—e.g. pleura and peritoneum), *purulent* (containing *pus*—numerous dead and dying bacteria, polymorphs and host tissue cells) and *haemorrhagic* (with many red cells).

Mediators

Many have been proposed but few proved. *Histamine*, released predominantly from local mast cells, is the principal mediator of the immediate response, and produces the initial arteriolar dilatation. The *kinins* (e.g. bradykinin) are derived from the circulation by a cascade system and are largely responsible for increased vascular permeability; they also maintain vasodilatation and produce local pain. Other substances possibly involved as mediators and/or chemotaxins include biologically active complement cleavage products (e.g. C3a, C5a and C567), extracts released from dead polymorphs (e.g. lysosomal enzymes), prostaglandins and fibrin products.

Spread

Usually, the acute inflammatory reaction succeeds in restricting the agent responsible. However, local spread may occur, particularly when bacteria capable of secreting local tissue-destroying enzymes (e.g. hyaluronidase) are responsible. In more severe cases, the agent may enter draining lymphatics and initiate acute inflammation in their walls (*acute lymphangitis*). Regional lymph nodes usually provide the next line of defence, and are probably involved to some extent in all episodes of acute inflammation. There is hyperplasia of germinal centres and sinusoidal histiocytes (*acute lymphadenitis* or *reactive hyperplasia*); if antigens are involved, the immune response is initiated (Chapter 6). When particulate matter, including bacteria and dead cells, enters the circulation, it is normally removed by the *mononuclear phagocyte (reticulo-endothelial) system* cells scattered in connective tissues throughout the body (histiocytes) and aggregated in certain organs, for example liver (Kupffer cells), bone marrow, spleen and lungs.

Results

If the inflammatory response destroys or neutralises the causative agent without significant local tissue damage, *resolution* (i.e. total restoration of normality) occurs. With tissue destruction, normality may be restored by local tissue proliferation (*regeneration*); if regeneration cannot occur, there will be *organisation* and replacement of damaged tissues by *fibrosis* (see 'Chronic Inflammation' below and Chapter 4). *Suppuration* (pus formation) may develop, with collections of pus producing *abscesses*. If the agent persists, *chronic inflammation* will supervene.

CHRONIC INFLAMMATION

Introduction

These changes, occurring over weeks, months or years, indicate a prolonged or persistent insult, and represent the body's attempt to localise the causative agent and to repair the resulting damage.

Causes

Chronic inflammation may follow acute inflammation (see above) or arise de novo. Common causes are listed in Table 3.2; some are discussed elsewhere—organisms (Chapter 5), cell-mediated hypersensitivity (Chapter 6) and poor blood supply (Chapter 8).

Table 3.2 Causes of chronic inflammation

Organisms—Bacteria, especially *Mycobacteria*
  —Treponema (syphilis)
  —Fungi
  —Parasites (e.g. *Schistosoma*)
Foreign material—Industrial—Silica
            —Asbestos
        —Sutures
        —Talc
Cell-mediated hypersensitivity—Tuberculosis
            —Sarcoidosis
            —Autoimmune diseases
Poor blood supply (e.g. varicose ulcers)
'Chemical' (e.g. peptic ulcers)
Persistence of agent causing acute inflammation

Cells involved

Cells involved may be from blood or local tissues.

Blood cells are *lymphocytes* and *plasma cells* (cf. neutrophil polymorphs in acute inflammation), and they provide local cellular and humoral immunological defence reactions (described in Chapter 6). *Macrophages*, as in acute inflammation, are phagocytic and remove local tissue debris; sometimes they may form *multinucleated giant cells*, probably by fusion. Occasionally, *eosinophil polymorphs* are also present, particularly in parasitic infections and hypersensitivity reactions.

Tissue cells are mainly proliferating *fibroblasts* and prominent *endothelial cells* lining capillaries; they are invariably found together and constitute *granulation tissue*. They appear initially around the periphery of the chronic inflammatory focus and grow towards its centre. The fibroblasts secrete collagen, elastin and ground substance. Ultimately, most cells and capillaries gradually disappear, leading to *fibrosis* (scar tissue formation); this repair process is designated *organisation* (see also Chapter 4).

Granulomatous chronic inflammation

This is a variant where *macrophages* predominate in multiple, small, discrete, concentric aggregates (*granulomata*) scattered throughout the tissue. They are usually associated with cell-mediated hypersensitivity reactions, fungal infections, parasitic infestations or aseptic foreign material. They comprise an avascular mass of macrophages, some of which form multinucleated giant cells, at the centre of which may be the causative agent or cellular necrosis; around this mass is a cuff of lymphocytes, often with granulation tissue and, in older lesions, fibrosis.

Results

Scar tissue is usually beneficial—it limits the causative agent and ultimately repairs local tissue deficiencies. Occasionally, excess fibrosis may cause deformity, obstruction or immobilization of organs and tissues.

DENTAL ASPECTS

Inflammatory diseases occupy much of every dental practitioner's working life. It is important, therefore, that dental students understand the basic principles involved and the ways they may be modified in dental and oral tissues.

Pulpitis

Pulpitis, dental pulp inflammation, is usually due to dental caries, and represents one pulp reaction to bacteria in dentinal tubules; occasionally, it is produced by physical cutting of dentine or chemicals used during cavity preparation. The sequential tissue changes are identical to those of inflammation elsewhere; the outcome, however, is often different because of the local pulpodentinal anatomy. The early changes are *hyperaemia* with pulp capillary dilatation and fluid exudate forma-

tion. Clinically, hyperaemic pulp is transiently painful to hot, cold or sweet fluids. If the dental caries is removed and tooth tissue restored, these changes are usually reversible.

Acute pulpitis. Here, the inflammatory process has progressed to neutrophil polymorph accumulation. This is usually seen first in the pulp horns where caries is most evident and bacterial products are most highly concentrated. Later, numerous polymorphs die and release their lysosomal enzymes, killing both pulp tissue and bacteria; the result is an abscess localised to the pulp horn. Eventually, the entire pulp may become involved and die. Clinically, the pulp remains painful to hot, cold and sweet stimuli, but the pain may last for a considerable time and may occur spontaneously when chemical mediator levels are high. Unlike acute inflammation elsewhere, established acute pulpitis is unlikely to resolve and usually progresses to total pulp necrosis. This is because the fluid exudate is confined within unyielding, intact dentine walls, and the resulting increased pressure interferes with normal blood flow and predisposes to vascular thrombosis; bacterial and polymorph enzymes destroy pulp tissue; inflamed tissues need more nutrients and oxygen, and even slight vascular impairment will produce ischaemia (Chapter 8).

Chronic pulpitis. This may occur when pulp irritation is mild but prolonged. Microscopically, typical chronic inflammation is seen, with dilated blood vessels, predominantly perivascular lymphocyte and plasma cell infiltration and increased fibrosis. Clinically, there may be vague, transient discomfort exacerbated by temperature changes. Should the irritant intensity increase, a typical acute pulpitis may ensue.

Open pulpitis. Occasionally, carious dentine breaks down to expose dental pulp to the oral cavity. Under these circumstances, the pulp can withstand acute inflammation without eventual necrosis as all inflammatory products pass freely into the saliva. Microscopically, the pulp consists of granulation tissue with numerous lymphocytes and plasma cells and a variable polymorph infiltrate. Open pulpitis is usually found in young patients with good pulp blood supply through wide root apices.

Pulpitis should not be regarded as a series of distinct clinical and pathological conditions but as a spectrum ranging from hyperaemia to suppuration; this would explain the common finding of pulps showing both acute and chronic inflammation.

Periapical bone inflammation

Periapical maxillary or mandibular bone is often inflamed by an extension of dental pulp inflammation.

Periapical abscess

Acute pulpitis may spread to apical periodontal tissues with abscess formation in adjacent bone. The affected area and involved tooth are tender to touch, the overlying mucosa is often congested and oedematous, and regional lymph nodes may be tender and enlarged. Usually, the pus tracks spontaneously through the bone and discharges into the mouth. Without treatment, repeated attacks may occur, producing a chronic abscess cavity.

Apical granuloma

Apical extension from chronic pulpitis causes osteoclastic bone resorption, some of which is enhanced by mediators of inflammation (e.g. prostaglandins), and replacement by granulation tissue containing lymphocytes and plasma cells. Macrophages are also present as either mononuclear cells or multinucleated giant cells. Occasionally, particulate material accidentally introduced into the periapical bone during root canal treatment may produce or exacerbate an apical granuloma. Acute inflammation and abscess formation may supervene if local tissue damage increases.

4

Healing

General features
Introduction
Regeneration
Organisation
Factors delaying healing

Specific healing
Skin
Bone fractures
Epithelium
Muscle
Cartilage
Nervous tissue

Dental aspects
Oral mucosal ulceration
Extraction sockets
Mandibular fractures

GENERAL FEATURES

Introduction

Healing is the replacement of dead cells by living cells or fibrous tissue, and occurs by *regeneration* or *organisation*; the ultimate result depends on the local balance between these two factors.

Regeneration

This is replacement by proliferation of surviving cells of the same type—thus it is only seen in tissues capable of mitotic activity. Some cells (e.g. epidermis, gastrointestinal epithelium and red blood cells) invariably regenerate; others (e.g. liver, renal tubule epithelium and thyroid) will regenerate under favourable circumstances; some (e.g. neurones and cardiac muscle) can not regenerate. Total restoration of structural and functional normality, usually encountered only when cell loss is minimal, is *resolution*.

Organisation

This is replacement by fibrosis. It occurs in fibrinous acute inflammatory exudates and chronic inflammation (Chapter 3), and in infarcts and thrombi (Chapter 8). It begins with digestion and removal of debris by *macrophages* and growth into the necrotic area of *granulation tissue* (*capillary loops* with prominent lining endothelial cells and large, plump *fibroblasts*) from adjacent connective tissues. Some inflammatory cells, both acute and chronic, are also usually present. As healing progresses, fibroblasts lay down collagen and

ground substance, and cellularity is reduced by the gradual disappearance of inflammatory cells, fibroblasts and capillaries. Ultimately, only avascular and acellular collagenous *scar tissue* remains.

Factors delaying healing

These may be local or general.

Local factors include poor blood supply, persistence of infection, retention of foreign materials and repeated local movement or trauma.

General factors. Collagen synthesis is defective in vitamin C, zinc or protein (especially sulphur-containing amino acid) deficiency states. Diabetes mellitus, by predisposing to infection and vascular disease, retards healing. Excess glucocorticoid hormones actively suppress inflammation and healing. In general, healing is slower in elderly patients.

SPECIFIC HEALING

Skin

Exact changes depend on whether the skin edges are in apposition.

Primary union (healing by first intention) occurs when the edges are in contact, as when held by sutures following surgical incisions. Immediate haemorrhage produces a fibrin-rich blood clot in the small gap and a mild acute inflammatory reaction is initiated. Macrophages and granulation tissue soon invade the area—the former to remove debris including fibrin, the latter to begin the process of organisation, which continues rapidly until a relatively small scar is produced. Meanwhile, the squamous epithelium of the adjacent overlying epidermis migrates and proliferates until continuity is restored.

Secondary union (healing by second intention) occurs with extensive local tissue loss. The wound contains fibrin and tissue debris, and may initially be covered by a scab. A brisk acute inflammatory reaction develops and granulation tissue begins to grow into the area from the periphery. Within the granulation tissue are myofibroblasts which, because of their ability to contract, help to decrease wound size and thus accelerate healing. Ultimately, a large, irregular scar is produced. Simultaneously, cells from the overlying epidermis migrate and proliferate below the scab until regeneration is complete; skin appendages do not reappear.

Bone fractures

A fracture is a break in the continuity of bone. As with skin wounds, there is immediate haemorrhage from severed blood vessels and, unless local infection is present, only mild acute inflammation is produced. By 24 hours, macrophages and granulation tissue start invading the area, and after about 1 week, specific bone-forming cells (osteoblasts) begin laying down new osteoid as an irregular meshwork which soon mineralises to form *woven bone* or *provisional callus*. This woven bone, which ultimately unites the fracture, is gradually replaced by regular lamellar bone (*definitive callus*) and remodelling restores normal bone shape.

Epithelium

Surface epithelium (e.g. epidermis and gastrointestinal, respiratory and urogenital epithelia) possesses excellent regeneration potential. Once the causative agent is removed, healing is rapid and total. Local defects representing foci of surface epithelial loss are known as *ulcers*.

Glandular epithelium will regenerate under favourable circumstances, as when the agent or factor causing the original necrosis is removed rapidly and when the organ's supporting connective tissue framework (e.g. liver and renal tubules) remains intact. Sometimes, specialised glands are replaced by simpler glands (e.g. in stomach), and a few (e.g. skin adnexal structures) can not regenerate.

Muscle

Striated muscle regeneration is often very limited, but may be extensive if endomysial and perimysial fibrous sheaths remain intact.

Smooth muscle and *cardiac muscle* are virtually incapable of regeneration.

Cartilage

Cartilage does not regenerate and heals by organisation, although fibrous tissue thus produced may be converted into fibrocartilage.

Nervous tissue

Central nervous system (CNS) nerve cells never regenerate; replacement is by glial fibrils from astrocytes (*gliosis*), a variant of organisation unique to the nervous system. CNS axons also do not regenerate.

Peripheral nerves will not regenerate if the cell body is destroyed, and replacement is again by gliosis; however, peripheral axonal damage will result in considerable regeneration, especially if endoneurial tubes are undamaged.

DENTAL ASPECTS

Oral mucosal ulceration

This is a frequent event, commonly due to physical or chemical agents (e.g. hot foods and drinks, sharp implements and 'aspirin burn'). These ulcers heal quickly, leaving clinically normal tissues. Even each bout of recurrent ulceration (Chapter 15), although very painful, heals rapidly and uneventfully. When ulceration is severe (as in major aphthous ulceration), healing is prolonged and involves fibrosis and scarring. Sometimes fibrosis may be extensive, for example when a cusp of a fractured lower molar tooth is continually ulcerating the tongue; in such cases, the lesion may resemble a carcinoma. As a rule, therefore, oral ulcers that fail to heal within 2 or

3 weeks should be biopsied for microscopic examination.

Extraction sockets

Extraction sockets, created by tooth removal, can be regarded as a form of bone fracture. Although the amount of bone exposed is quite considerable, it is remarkable how effective healing is, as failure to heal is uncommon. Inadequate healing usually involves breakdown of blood clot in the socket and infection of devitalised bone by microorganisms. When teeth are extracted from bone with an excessive or a poor blood supply (e.g. Paget's disease), such infected sockets ('dry sockets') are more common, and although bone healing is usually rapid and the integrity of the oral mucosa quickly restored, final remodelling within the socket can take many months; this is indicated radiographically by persistence of lamina dura.

Mandibular fractures

In elderly patients, mandibular blood supply from the inferior dental artery is reduced, most of the blood coming from periosteal vessels. This will delay healing of mandibular fractures, and emphasises the necessity to avoid raising periosteal flaps during splinting procedures.

5

Infections

Introduction
General features
Microorganism factors
Host factors
Results of infection
Some specific infections
Introduction
Bacteria

Viruses
Spirochaetes
Rickettsiae
Chlamydiae
Mycoplasmas
Fungi and yeasts
Protozoa
Dental examples

INTRODUCTION

Numerous microorganisms, including bacteria, viruses, spirochaetes, rickettsiae, chlamydiae, mycoplasmas, fungi, yeasts and protozoa, can infect the human body. Some of these (e.g. on the skin) are present normally and are harmless (*commensals*); a few (e.g. in the bowel) may even benefit the host (*saprophytes*). Many, however, are *pathogenic*—that is, they cause disease by damaging host cells and tissues. These distinctions, although helpful, are not rigid; under certain circumstances (e.g. immunosuppression), commensal organisms may become pathogenic, producing *opportunistic infections*.

GENERAL FEATURES

The type, extent and severity of damage produced by any pathogenic microorganism are influenced by numerous factors prevailing at the time of infection. Some of these are considered briefly below, and relate to either organism or host factors.

Microorganism factors

Access. In order to cause disease, organisms must gain access to body cells and tissues, and most enter via respiratory or gastrointestinal tracts. Commensals may become pathogens when they are transferred to other sites—for example *Streptococcus viridans* entering the circulation may cause endocarditis; *Escherichia coli* in the urinary tract may cause cystitis.

Dose and virulence. Dose indicates the number of organisms entering the body and virulence reflects their capacity to cause disease. In general, the larger the dose, the greater is the likelihood of disease becoming established, but the higher their virulence, the fewer organisms are required. Within species, different strains may show differences in virulence.

Invasiveness. This indicates ability to multiply and spread. Invasion is facilitated by endotoxin and extracellular enzyme production: *endotoxins*, intimately associated with organism cell walls, are liberated on autolysis to produce host tissue cell damage; *extracellular enzymes* (e.g. coagulase, collagenase and hyaluronidase) digest local tissues and protect the organisms from body defence mechanisms. In addition, *exotoxins*, secreted by organisms into their environment, may produce distant or generalised toxic effects.

Transmission. Long term survival of any microorganism depends on its ability to pass to another suitable host. Thus, many are transmitted via droplets from the respiratory tract or via faeces; several form resistant spores; some require specific intermediate animal vectors; a few need close physical contact.

Host factors

Most are non-specific and designed to prevent infection by a range of pathogenic microorganisms; in contrast, immunological responses are aimed at specific invading organisms.

Physical barriers. Intact skin and mucous membranes of respiratory, alimentary and urinary tracts provide important barriers to infection, and

15

many pathogens require defects in these tissues to gain access. In addition, the skin and many mucosal surfaces are normally covered by numerous commensals which help to oppose the establishment of pathogenic organisms.

Physiological barriers. Many of these prevent pathogens gaining access, and include mucous secretion and ciliary action in the respiratory tract, secretions on the skin, salivary enzymes in the mouth and acidic pH in the stomach. When pathogens enter the circulation, they are normally removed by the mononuclear phagocyte (reticuloendothelial) system cells scattered throughout the body in connective tissue and aggregated in certain organs, for example liver, bone marrow, spleen and lungs.

Inflammatory response. Pathogenic organisms are the main causes of acute and chronic inflammation, and the inflammatory response is one of the most important of the body's natural defence mechanisms (Chapter 3).

Immunological responses. These provide resistance to and immunity against specific infecting agents (Chapter 6).

Local factors. Certain features at the site of pathogen entry (e.g. ischaemia and persistent foreign material) will promote infection and impair eradication. Some organisms (e.g. *Clostridia*) are anaerobic, and thus require local hypoxia.

Systemic factors. Several systemic conditions or diseases predispose to infections; these include malnutrition (especially protein and vitamin C deficiencies), chronic alcoholism, diabetes mellitus, Cushing's syndrome and generalised debilitated states such as disseminated malignant disease and chronic renal failure.

Age. Both the very young and the very old have an increased susceptibility to infectious diseases.

Drugs. Appropriate antimicrobial drugs in adequate blood concentrations help to eradicate many susceptible microorganisms.

Results of infection

The outcome of any pathogenic microorganism infection is invariably one of the following:

Eradication. Fortunately, most infections end in total eradication of the organisms at the point of entry. Associated clinical signs and symptoms vary from very mild to severe; occasionally, the whole process is asymptomatic (i.e. an inapparent infection).

Persistence. A few organisms, having entered the body, may persist for many years. The infected individuals may be asymptomatic carriers (e.g. typhoid bacillus and hepatitis B virus); they may develop repeated acute attacks (e.g. herpes virus); they may have continuous chronic inflammation (e.g. staphylococcal chronic osteomyelitis); they may have progressive and ultimately fatal disease (e.g. hepatitis B virus).

Spread. Pathogenic organisms may spread locally, helped largely by endotoxin or extracellular enzyme production (see 'Invasiveness of Microorganisms' above). Further spread may occur—to regional lymph nodes, through coelomic cavities (e.g. pleura and peritoneum) or via the blood stream. Haematogenous dissemination may be as *bacteraemia* (i.e. organisms in the blood), *septicaemia* (i.e. actively multiplying organisms in the blood) or *pyaemia* (i.e. groups of pyogenic organisms in the blood).

Host death. Occasionally, infections may result in host death; more than one type of organism may be responsible, and invariably one or more adverse host factors (see above) apply. Usually, the normal body defence mechanisms are overwhelmed, but sometimes death is due to exotoxin production (e.g. tetanus and diphtheria).

SOME SPECIFIC INFECTIONS

Introduction

Characteristics of pathogenic microorganisms and their classifications are the province of microbiologists, and are considered in appropriate microbiology textbooks.

In the remainder of this chapter, some specific infections are discussed, and others, described later with the relevant organ or system, are mentioned.

Bacteria

Bacteria are the commonest cause of acute inflammation. Many (e.g. staphylococci, streptococci and coliforms) are *pyogenic*—that is they are associated with *pus* and *abscess* formation. A few (e.g. *Mycobacteria*) elicit a chronic inflammatory response. Several are described elsewhere—for example pneumococcus, Chapter 14; meningococcus, Chapter 24; gonococcus, Chapter 18; *Clostridium welchii*, Chapter 2.

Tuberculosis

Tuberculosis is infection by *Mycobacterium tuberculosis*. It is a very important, widespread, endemic disease which can develop at any age. Although there has been a marked decrease in its incidence and mortality in the last 50 years, particularly in more developed countries, it still affects over 50 million individuals worldwide and kills 5 million annually.

Transmission. Four possible entry sites exist—respiratory tract and oropharyngeal lymphoid tissue by inhalation, alimentary tract by ingestion and skin by innoculation; 'congenital' infection following intra-uterine transmission from a tuberculous placenta is very rare. Entry via the alimentary tract is now uncommon in countries where bovine tuberculosis has been eradicated and heat treatment of milk is routine, and most infection is by droplet spread and inhalation from active 'open cases'.

Pathogenesis. This is influenced by organism and host factors as discussed above.

Pathology. Tuberculosis usually affects the lungs, but may involve any organ or tissue. It produces a granulomatous chronic inflammatory response; the granulomata, sometimes designated tubercles, usually have a central area of amorphous, acellular *caseous* necrosis, and consist mainly of macrophages, sometimes referred to as *epithelioid cells*. Some macrophages fuse to form multinucleated giant cells, the nuclei of which may be distributed peripherally (i.e. classical *Langhans' giant cells*). Excessive caseation produces a *cold abscess*, so called because there is no associated acute inflammation. Healing, when present, is by progressive fibrosis, but organisms may remain viable in apparently healed lesions only to be reactivated years later if host resistance decreases.

Spread. Organisms may spread from the entry site in the usual ways—locally into adjacent tissues, by lymphatics to regional lymph nodes, along natural passages (e.g. respiratory, alimentary, urinary and genital tracts) and via the blood to produce either *miliary tuberculosis*, with multiple tubercles in numerous organs and tissues, or single organ disease.

Immunology. The granulomatous reaction indicates a cell-mediated (type IV) immunological response (Chapter 6) to an antigenic protein component of the organism (*tuberculoprotein*). This response produces the basis of several diagnostic skin tests (e.g. Mantoux) and can be induced artificially by injecting attenuated mycobacterial strains (e.g. BCG).

Primary tuberculosis. This follows initial exposure in non-immunised individuals of any age. There is usually a small tuberculous focus at the entry site, and, because immunity is absent, numerous organisms spread rapidly to regional lymph nodes producing marked tuberculous nodal enlargement. This small parenchymal focus (which in the lung is often called the *Ghon focus*) and the considerably enlarged regional lymph nodes are usually designated the *primary complex*. Once immunity has developed, healing by fibrosis without further spread is usual, and the primary infection is invariably asymptomatic; however, haematogenous dissemination occurs most commonly at this stage, producing either miliary tuberculosis or single organ involvement which may become clinically apparent later.

Secondary (reinfection) tuberculosis. This follows reactivation of the primary infection or represents infection of an individual previously immunised either naturally by prior exposure or artificially by BCG; in patients under 40 years of age it is usually *endogenous* (i.e. reactivation), whereas over that age it is probably *exogenous* (i.e. reinfection). For secondary tuberculosis to become established, there is often some impairment of normal immune mechanisms, and one or more adverse host factors described earlier in this chapter may apply. In secondary tuberculosis, parenchymal damage is usually marked, with minimal regional lymph node involvement (cf. primary tuberculosis); the lung is the commonest organ involved, and characteristically, the lesions are confined to one or both apices. It may heal by fibrosis with scarring or may spread (see above).

Treatment. Appropriate antituberculous drugs in adequate dosage over several months will modify the disease and help to eradicate the organisms.

Definitive diagnosis. This depends on demonstration of organisms in relevant specimens (e.g. sputum, urine and tissues after biopsy) by Ziehl–Neelsen staining, bacteriological culture or guinea pig inoculation. Positive skin tests (e.g. Mantoux) merely indicate hypersensitivity to tuberculoprotein; they do not indicate active disease, and may even be negative in overwhelming, severe tuberculosis.

Leprosy

Leprosy is caused by *Mycobacterium leprae*. It is a very indolent and prolonged infection requiring many years of close contact for transmission and a long (perhaps 5–10 years) incubation period. The organism elicits a cell-mediated (type IV) immunological reaction, the extent of which determines the form of leprosy produced.

Lepromatous leprosy occurs in less resistant patients. They develop multiple skin, subcutaneous, oral and nasal aggregates of macrophages containing numerous lepra bacilli.

Tuberculoid leprosy occurs in more resistant hosts. They develop tubercle-like nodules without caseation and lepra bacilli are fewer. Skin and peripheral nerves are involved early, and sensory loss is common.

Actinomycosis

Actinomycosis is caused by *Actinomyces israelii*, a virtually anaerobic organism, classified as a bacterium despite possessing branching hyphae (cf. fungi below), which is sometimes found as a commensal in the mouth and alimentary tract. Occasionally, it may become pathogenic and, as it is more common in cattle, farm workers are more liable to the disease. In almost 70% of cases the lower face and neck are involved; in about 15% the infection is intestinal (often around the ileocaecal region or appendix); in about 10% multiple pulmonary lesions follow inhalation; about 5% develop subcutaneous lesions. Actinomycosis produces firm masses containing numerous abscesses bearing organism colonies as yellowish granules ('*sulphur granules*'); considerable local tissue destruction occurs, and sinuses and fistulae are common. Histologically, there is granulomatous chronic inflammation with suppuration (i.e. polymorphs producing pus). Rarely, organisms enter the circulation, and similar abscesses may develop throughout the body.

Viruses

Viruses are relatively simple, small, obligatory parasites which replicate within cells by synthesis and assembly of separate components rather than by division, and which are entirely dependent on host cell metabolism for survival and replication. Viruses damage the cells in which they live, and often cause cell death; they frequently produce intracytoplasmic or intranuclear eosinophilic inclusions and may elicit a variable, often mild chronic inflammatory reaction. Most viral infections are transient and not severe, with subsequent total recovery and immunity against the specific strain involved (e.g. common cold and influenza); occasionally, the initial infection is asymptomatic, but spread causes subsequent disease (e.g. poliomyelitis); rarely, the infection is severe and fatal (e.g. smallpox and rabies). A few viruses may persist for many years (e.g. herpes simplex and varicella). Recently *slow viruses*, with incubation periods of several years and producing prolonged disease, have aroused interest, particularly in certain cerebral diseases (Chapter 24). Several specific viral infections are described elsewhere, for example hepatitis A and B (Chapter 17); glandular fever (infectious mononucleosis), Chapter 21; viruses causing mucocutaneous lesions (Chapter 25). Viruses related to neoplasia are considered in Chapter 10.

Mumps is an acute, contagious viral infection usually encountered in childhood. Over 90% of patients develop painful parotid swelling, which is usually bilateral. In about 10% of cases, one or more other major salivary gland is involved, and about 20% of males develop orchitis (inflammation of the testis), usually unilateral. Less commonly, spread to other organs (e.g. pancreas, ovaries, meninges and brain) also occurs. Affected tissues show interstitial oedema and infiltration by lymphocytes, plasma cells and macrophages, with variable, mild epithelial cell degeneration and necrosis; polymorphs are uncommon and infrequent. The lesions usually heal rapidly after 1–2 weeks with minimal residual fibrosis and atrophy.

Spirochaetes

Spirochaetes are actively motile, coiled, unicellular spiral-shaped organisms which usually produce interstitial chronic inflammation with predominantly perivascular plasma cell, lymphocyte and macrophage aggregation.

Syphilis

Syphilis is infection by *Treponema pallidum*. Over the last 25 years its incidence has undoubtedly increased.

Transmission. The organism is very vulnerable to drying, and must be acquired by close physical contact; this contact is invariably sexual, hence syphilis is a venereal disease. As the organism is probably unable to penetrate intact epidermis, a minor, possibly microscopic, abrasion is necessary for transmission. Occasionally, syphilis is congenital (see below). Characteristically, three stages of acquired syphilis are described, although progression is not inevitable and any stage may be asymptomatic; furthermore, early adequate and appropriate antimicrobial drug treatment may eradicate the organism and prevent progression.

Primary syphilis. Although there is organism dissemination throughout the body within 24 hours of infection, the primary lesion does not develop for 1–6 (usually 3–4) weeks, and is confined to the entry site and regional lymph nodes. This site is genital (i.e. penis in males and vulva or cervix in females) in about 90% of cases; possible non-genital sites include rectum, lips, mouth, fingers and breasts. The primary lesion (*chancre*) is a solitary, slowly enlarging, hard, usually painless nodule which soon shows superficial ulceration. Histologically, there is intense chronic inflammation with granulation tissue formation at the periphery; polymorphs indicate secondary bacterial invasion, which is fairly common. The enlarged regional lymph nodes are often painless, and show lymphadenitis (Chapter 3). With or without treatment, the chancre heals after several weeks with minimal residual scar tissue; it may pass undetected, especially if on the uterine cervix, and sometimes may never develop clinically.

Secondary syphilis. Some manifestations develop in most untreated patients, usually 1–3 months after infection. These are numerous, and may include skin rashes (usually maculopapular and often involving palms and soles), shallow buccal, lingual and pharyngeal ulceration ('*snail-track*' *ulcers*), flat, slightly elevated papules on external genitalia (*condylomata lata*), scalp hair follicle involvement causing loss of hair (*alopecia*), generalised lymph node enlargement and non-specific features such as malaise, pyrexia, anorexia and anaemia. Again, with or without treatment, these lesions disappear gradually over several months. About one-third of these patients, even if untreated, show spontaneous 'cure', and serological tests (see below) become negative; about one-third remain seropositive, but do not develop further disease; the remainder progress to tertiary syphilis.

Tertiary syphilis. This appears several (usually 5–30) years after primary infection, but may well be asymptomatic. In most patients, the cardiovascular system is involved, with chronic inflammatory weakening of the ascending aortic wall producing aneurysmal dilatation, aortic incompetence and coronary ostia narrowing (Chapter 12); in 5–10%, CNS involvement produces meningovascular disease, general paralysis of the insane or tabes dorsalis (Chapter 24); the remainder have one or more gummas, which may be from a few millimetres to several centimetres in diameter. A *gumma* is a firm, rubbery, nodular mass; it may be found anywhere in the body, but especially in liver, bones and testes. Extensive tissue destruction, with overlying epithelial ulceration, is usual. Histologically, gummas show considerable central avascular and acellular coagulative necrosis surrounded by granulation tissue containing numerous chronic inflammatory cells, particularly plasma cells; more peripherally, collagen is deposited, with blood vessels showing intimal thickening and proliferation (*endarteritis obliterans*) and perivascular aggregates of plasma cells and lymphocytes; giant cells are infrequent and polymorphs are usually absent. With time, healing by fibrosis can occur spontaneously, but this is much more likely after adequate chemotherapy. Gummas may be asymptomatic or of little clinical importance, but the associated local tissue destruction can produce severe clinical symptoms.

Congenital syphilis. This is due to transplacental spread; it is now uncommon in countries where serological screening (see below) is performed routinely on all pregnant women. Extent and severity of fetal infection dictate outcome in the offspring—thus, there may be late abortion, stillbirth, neonatal death or disease presenting in infancy, childhood or even adult life. Manifestations are numerous and diverse: in infancy, they include desquamating skin rashes (particularly on palms, soles, face and buttocks), osteochondritis (especially of nasal bones producing saddle deformity, 'snuffles' and impaired feeding), epiphysitis (causing irregular ossification and bone deformities), diffuse hepatic fibrosis, diffuse interstitial pulmonary fibrosis and chronic meningitis; in later childhood and early adulthood there may be permanent dentition abnormalities (Hutchinson's peg-shaped incisors with notched edges or Moon's dome-shaped and pitted molars), interstitial keratitis causing corneal opacity and blindness, periostitis causing bone deformities (e.g. 'sabre tibia'), one or more gummas and central nervous system involvement (as in acquired tertiary syphilis).

Immunology. Syphilitic infection induces antibodies which may be detected in the serum by well-established techiques—for example Wasserman reaction (WR), Kahn and VDRL (venereal disease research laboratory) tests. These are useful screening techniques, but positivity takes several weeks to develop, and they may become negative, even in untreated latent cases; furthermore, false positive reactions can occur (e.g. in untreated systemic lupus erythematosus, glandular fever and malaria). A much more specific antibody reaction is the treponemal immobilization test (TPI), where the patient's serum causes immobilization of viable treponemes.

Definitive diagnosis. This requires either demonstration of specific serum antibodies (above) or identification of causative organisms in affected tissues. The organisms may be seen, although with difficulty, in smears or histological sections; more recently, they have been identified by specific fluorescent antibody methods.

Rickettsiae

Rickettsiae are obligatory intracellular parasites, smaller than bacteria, which require exogenous energy for their growth. They are endemic in many animals and birds, and transmission to humans of all except one depends on arthropod vectors (e.g. lice, fleas, ticks and mites); the exception is *Coxiella burnetii* causing Q fever (see below). Rickettsiae disseminate throughout the body soon after entry, preferentially colonise small blood vessel endothelium and produce vascular swelling or thrombosis with consequent ischaemia and infarction; they elicit a variable inflammatory cell reaction comprising polymorphs, lymphocytes, plasma cells and macrophages. Rickettsiae cause epidemic and endemic *typhus*, common throughout the world but very rare in this country, and Q fever, which is occasionally encountered here.

Q fever is mainly a disease of farm animals, but may spread to humans by droplet inhalation or ingestion. It usually causes an atypical pneumonia, but may produce severe subacute infective endocarditis (Chapter 13).

Chlamydiae

Chlamydiae are also small, obligatory intracellular parasites, but possess two forms—one for intracellular multiplication, the other, a spore-like body, for extracellular survival. In humans, chlamydiae elicit both humoral and cell-mediated immunity; the latter produces the usual granulomatous chronic inflammatory response. Chlamydial infections include *ornithosis* (an atypical pneumonia following inhalation from faeces of infected birds, particularly parrots and budgerigars), *trachoma* (conjunctival inflammation leading to scarring and blindness—Chapter 24) and *lymphogranuloma inguinale* (a venereal disease with a small ulcerated genital lesion and marked regional lymph node enlargement produced by numerous granulomas; necrosis with abscess formation is extensive).

Mycoplasmas

Mycoplasmas are the smallest free-living cells known; they lack cell walls, but can replicate in cell free environments and may be cultured, albeit slowly, in laboratories. Although responsible for many plant and animal diseases, only one is definitely pathogenic for humans—*Mycoplasma pneumoniae* produces a relatively mild atypical pneumonia and elicits a predominantly chronic inflammatory reaction.

Fungi and yeasts

Fungi consist of filaments (*hyphae*) which grow by continuous extension and branching, and which produce spores; *yeasts* are single, oval or spherical cells which multiply by budding. However, this distinction is not absolute, as several organisms can exist as either form, depending on environmental circumstances. Numerous fungi and yeasts are known, but very few are pathogenic to humans; most cause trivial and superficial infections (e.g. athlete's foot), but some may produce more severe and occasionally fatal systemic disease, particularly in immune deficient or immunosuppressed patients. The associated inflammatory reaction is extremely variable, and depends on nature, site and extent of infection and integrity of host immune and inflammatory responses—thus mild superficial infections elicit mild chronic inflammation, whereas severe systemic disease may show both acute and chronic inflammation with necrosis and abscess formation; some fungi induce the granulomatous variant.

Candidosis (moniliasis)

This is due to *Candida albicans*, a normal commensal of moist skin, mouth and intestines. Superficial invasion usually produces disease, particularly in skin creases, oral mucosa, oesophagus and vagina. Systemic disease, following haematogenous dissemination, is rare, and results in multiple, small abscesses.

Cryptococcosis

This is due to *Cryptococcus neoformans*, and often follows its inhalation from the faeces of infected birds, particularly pigeons. It may remain localised to the lungs, where it causes granulomatous inflammation, or may spread to other organs, particularly meninges.

Histoplasmosis

This is due to *Histoplasma capsulatum*. Its spores are present in animal and bird faeces and often enter humans by inhalation. Asymptomatic mild pulmonary inflammation is usual, but dissemination may occur—organisms proliferate within macrophages and there is particular involvement of spleen, liver, lymph nodes, bone marrow and lungs, invariably with granuloma formation and necrosis.

Aspergillosis

Many *Aspergillus* species exist, but the only important human pathogen is *Aspergillus fumigatus*. It is almost always inhaled, thus causing such lung diseases as asthma and pneumonia; haematogenous dissemination may occur, but is very rare.

Protozoa

Protozoa, although relatively uncommon in temperate climates, are important and frequent causes of disease worldwide. Many protozoal infections exist, including *leishmaniasis* (spread by sandflies), *trypanosomiasis* (spread by tsetse flies or cone-nosed bugs) and *amoebiasis* (probably transmitted from person to person), but only two, malaria and toxoplasmosis, are considered briefly below.

Malaria

Malaria is common in many tropical and subtropical areas, but is encountered only occasionally in immigrants and travellers in this country. The genus *Plasmodium* is responsible, with different species (*falciparum*, *vivax*, *ovale* and *malariae*) producing different clinical manifestations. Anopheles mosquitoes provide the definitive host whilst vertebrates, including humans, are intermediate hosts. In humans, the parasites pass via the blood stream from the point of entry to the liver, from which, after maturation, they enter erythrocytes. Here, they develop further and multiply asexually; ultimately, infected red cells rupture and parasites re-enter the circulation to invade other erythrocytes to repeat the whole cycle.

Signs and symptoms. These are varied and include haemolytic anaemia (from red cell destruction—Chapter 20), pyrexia (coinciding with parasite release from erythrocytes), mononuclear phagocyte system hyperplasia (especially in spleen, liver and lymph nodes), multiple small cerebral infarcts (due to vascular occlusion by damaged red cells) and haemoglobinuria ('blackwater fever').

Results. These are obviously influenced by appropriate drug treatment. There may be a fairly short acute illness with progression to death or subsequent cure; usually, some resistance develops, and the infection becomes chronic, with numerous superadded acute exacerbations.

Toxoplasmosis

Toxoplasmosis, due to *Toxoplasma gondii*, may cause congenital or acquired disease, but is usually asymptomatic.

Congenital toxoplasmosis follows transplacental spread from an infected, but often symptomless, mother. Results include abortion, stillbirth, an infant with severe abnormalities (e.g. cerebral necrosis, hydrocephalus or blindness) or a normal infant which soon develops mild features of acquired disease.

Acquired toxoplasmosis probably results from food contamination by faeces of domestic pets, particularly cats. The commonest symptoms, when present, are lymph node enlargement (due to excess macrophage-like cells) and pyrexia; other organs (e.g. lungs, brain, eyes and heart) are rarely involved. Organism isolation is difficult and unreliable; rising antibody titres are usually used to confirm the diagnosis.

DENTAL EXAMPLES

Oral infections cover a wide spectrum, including the extremely common conditions of dental caries and periodontal disease (discussed in Chapters 6 and 15). Other common infections encountered in dental practice are:

Herpes simplex. Herpes simplex virus (HSV) type I is a DNA-containing virus with an affinity, in the adult, for epithelial tissues. It produces oral ulceration and 'cold sores' on the lips. Rarely, in young children, widespread dissemination may be followed by severe illness and death.

Primary infection is usually subclinical; in a few patients, however, there is vesiculation followed by painful oral and lip ulceration, bleeding and inflamed gingivae, cervical lymphadenopathy, fever and malaise (*herpetic gingivostomatitis*). Tissue scraped from the vesicles shows multinucleated epithelial cells and cells with dispersed chromatin (ballooning degenerating cells). Although typically a disease of childhood, it is now not uncommon to find adults with herpetic gingivostomatitis. Patients recover quickly, but may have recurrent attacks, often induced by unrelated illness or exposure to sunlight.

Recurrent infections are caused by re-activation of the virus which, following primary infection, is not eradicated but remains dormant within trigeminal nerves and ganglia. Intra-oral ulceration may develop, but the hallmark of recurrent infection is the ulcerated, crusted, 'cold sore' on the lip (*herpes labialis*). It is possible for dental surgeons to acquire lesions on the fingers ('herpetic whitlow') from contact with an infected patient.

Herpe zoster (shingles). The varicella–zoster virus causes chickenpox and shingles. The latter is a painful infection of dorsal root and cranial nerve (usually trigeminal) ganglia. Painful skin erythema of the affected dermatome with ulceration is typical; oral ulceration may be present, but, unlike herpes simplex, only one side of the mouth is affected. The pain can be intense, and may mimic toothache. Elderly patients are susceptible to prolonged postherpetic neuralgia following clinical resolution of the zoster. Involvement of the first branch of the trigeminal nerve may lead to corneal ulceration, which, if untreated, can lead to blindness.

Candidosis. Oral infection by *Candida albicans*, an opportunistic pathogen, is common. There are several clinical presentations, including *chronic atrophic candidosis* (a red 'soggy' appearance of palatal epithelium, covered by dentures, which may or may not be painful), *acute pseudomembranous candidosis* ('thrush'), *acute atrophic candidosis* (a sore mouth following suppression of oral commensal bacteria by antibiotics), *candidal leukoplakia* (a premalignant white patch induced by *Candida*) and *median rhomboid glossitis* of the tongue. Diagnosis in each case is on clinical grounds, and hyphal forms of *Candida* are often identified in smears taken from abnormal areas. Recurrent infections may develop in patients with endocrine, immunological or haematological abnormalities. *C. albicans*, as well as *Staphylococcus aureus*, may cause *angular cheilitis*—the red eroded or fissured lines at the angles of the mouth common in denture wearers.

6

Immunopathology

Introduction
Definitions
Cells of the immune system
Antibodies
Functions
Types
Sequence of production
Hapten recognition

Immunity
Lymphokines
Complement activation
Classical pathway
Alternate pathway
Immunodeficient states
Primary
Secondary

Hypersensitivity reactions
HLA system
Functions
Autoimmune diseases
Graft reactions
Dental aspects

INTRODUCTION

Knowledge of the immune system has progressed so rapidly recently that many diseases are now recognised as having an immunopathological basis. Accordingly, it is important for the student to appreciate, in some detail, the cellular interactions of the immune system and some of the ways in which it can produce disease.

DEFINITIONS

Antigen—A substance capable of evoking an immune response.
Antibody—A protein (immunoglobulin) produced by plasma cells in response to antigenic stimulation of the B lymphocyte system (humoral immunity). Antibodies bind in a specific manner to antigens.
Lymphokine—A soluble substance produced *mainly* by T lymphocytes in response to antigenic stimulation (cell-mediated immunity). Lymphokines do not bind to antigens.
Hapten—A substance which is not antigenic by itself but which is capable of binding to another molecule to form an antigen.
Autoimmune reaction—An abnormal immune response against the body's own tissues.
Hypersensitivity reactions—A group of immunological responses damaging body tissues.
Tolerance—A state of refractoriness where antigen introduction does not evoke an immune response.
Autograft—Tissue transplanted to another site in the same individual.

Homograft—Tissue transplanted between individuals of the same species:
(a) *syngeneic*—donor and recipient are genetically identical.
(b) *allogeneic*—donor and recipient are not genetically identical.
Heterograft (xenograft)—Tissue transplanted from one species to another.

CELLS OF THE IMMUNE SYSTEM

The formative tissues of the immune system are lymph nodes, spleen, bone marrow and thymus, but ultimately it is the haemopoietic stem cells which give rise to the individual cell types.

B lymphocytes are found in bone marrow, lymphoid follicles and splenic white pulp, and constitute 10–20% of peripheral blood lymphocytes. Their name is derived from the Bursa of Fabricius, the organ in birds responsible for their production; its removal causes a total loss of B cell function, although T cell activity is unchanged. They express cell surface IgM and IgD (below) which bind antigens, resulting in their clonal expansion by proliferation as B immunoblasts, some of which go on to form B memory cells, the remainder differentiating into antibody-producing plasma cells (Fig. 6.1). Memory cells are responsible for the rapid onset of the secondary antibody response (below).

T lymphocytes are so called because they require the thymus in infancy for correct functioning. Hence, thymectomised animals are deficient in T

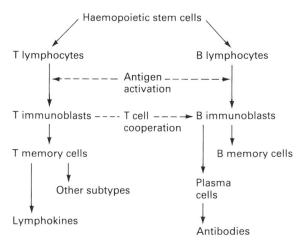

Fig. 6.1 Lymphocyte differentiation in the immune system

cell number and activity. T lymphocytes comprise 80–90% of peripheral blood lymphocytes, and are also found in paracortical areas of lymph nodes. Their activation (Fig. 6.1) is similar to that for B lymphocytes. They possess much less surface immunoglobulin, but have other surface receptors for antigens. In addition to lymphokine–producing and memory T cells, several subtypes exist:

Helper T cells augment B cell responses; without them, antibody production is impaired.
Suppressor T cells also interact with B cells but inhibit antibody production.
Contra suppressor T cells inhibit suppressor T cells.
Cytotoxic T cells play a role in killing, by direct membrane contact, virus-infected and neoplastic cells and in graft rejection.

Clearly, therefore, T cells play an important role in modulating immune responses, in defence against virus-infected cells, in graft rejection, in immune surveillance and in delayed hypersensitivity (tissue reaction to lymphokines).
Killer cells (K cells) lack surface markers of T and B lymphocytes but carry receptors for the Fc portion of immunoglobulins (below). They play a role in type II hypersensitivity reactions and in destruction of tumour cells. They are antibody-dependent cytotoxic cells (ADCC), that is their cytotoxicity depends on target cells reacting with antibodies (unlike cytotoxic T cells) to which the K cells in turn bind via their Fc receptors. This antibody-mediated contact leads to target cell death.

Natural killer cells (NK cells) lack both surface markers of T and B lymphocytes and Fc receptors. They play a role in immunosurveillance against neoplastic and virus-infected cells. It is uncertain whether they represent a distinct cell lineage or are members of the T lymphocyte series. Target cell killing involves cell to cell contact but, unlike ADCC, does not require antibody.

Macrophages, in addition to scavenging, have several roles:

1. Trapping, processing and transferring of antigens to lymphocytes.
2. Modulating lymphocyte activity.
3. Killing by ADCC, as they have surface Fc receptors.
4. Production of interferon and prostaglandins, which may allow them to modulate NK cell activity.
5. Synthesis of complement components.
6. Modulation of haemopoiesis.
7. Secretion of enzymes, e.g. collagenase.

They can be activated by lymphokines, complement by-products, antigen-antibody complexes and bacterial lipopolysaccharides.

ANTIBODIES

Antibodies comprise five immunoglobulin classes with characteristic heavy chains—α in IgA, δ in IgD, ϵ in IgE, γ in IgG and μ in IgM. Each antibody has two identical heavy chains and either kappa (κ) or lambda (λ) light chains, but never both. Each antibody has antibody-binding (Fab) and crystallisable (Fc) fragments. As a single plasma cell produces only one type of immunoglobulin, an infiltrate of plasma cells producing only one class of heavy and light chains is monoclonal and neoplastic (myeloma); an infiltrate producing both light chains and more than one heavy chain is polyclonal and non-neoplastic. All chains have a constant amino acid sequence and a variable region (Fig. 6.2); the latter permits antibody diversity so that no matter what the antigen, a specific antibody can be produced against it.

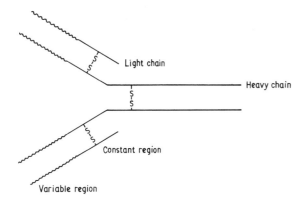

Fig. 6.2 Structure of immunoglobulins

Antibody functions

Irrespective of class, antibodies can be designated according to their main use; neutralising antibodies counteract toxins, opsonins coat bacteria to aid phagocytosis, complement-fixing antibodies activate complement and agglutinins bind bacteria together.

Types

IgA is the main antibody in saliva. In serum it is monomeric; in saliva it is dimeric, linked by a secretory protein. It hinders bacterial adherence to oral, pharyngeal and gastrointestinal epithelia.

IgD acts as antigen receptor on the surface of lymphocytes.

IgE is present in very small amounts in serum, and participates in type I hypersensitivity reactions.

IgG accounts for 75% of circulating immunoglobulins; it provides the major defence against microorganisms and toxins, produces natural passive immunity in the newborn (by passing across the placenta) and activates complement.

IgM is the first antibody secreted in response to antigenic stimulation. It is short lived, and the continued presence of antigen causes a switch in antibody class to IgG. A pentamer, linked by a J chain, it is a large molecule (molecular weight 900 000) and an efficient activator of complement.

Sequence of antibody production

A delay of several days or weeks exists between introduction of antigen into the body and detection of specific immunoglobulin in the blood. Initially, this is mainly IgM, the levels of which rise slightly before falling within 1–2 months (*primary antibody response*). Future antigen administration quickly produces immunoglobulin, mainly IgG; levels reached are high, and they fall slowly with time (*secondary antibody response*). Memory cells primed by the first antigen dose are responsible for the rapid and efficient antibody production of this secondary response.

Hapten recognition requires T and B lymphocyte cooperation. The carrier protein is recognised by T lymphocytes and the hapten by B lymphocytes. Examples include drugs such as penicillin which may bind to skin proteins to become antigenic.

IMMUNITY

Immunity against disease can be achieved in different ways:

Natural active immunity is obtained during the disease itself by the natural production of antibodies which will, in many instances, prevent subsequent attacks. Examples include most viral and bacterial infections.

Artificial active immunity is obtained by injecting attenuated infecting agents or toxins (i.e. toxoids) so that the immune system produces antibodies in the absence of actual disease. Examples include smallpox, tuberculosis (as BCG) and diphtheria.

Natural passive immunity is seen in infants who obtain antibodies via the placenta or their mothers' milk.

Acquired passive immunity follows administration of antibodies from another individual or species. To prevent tetanus, antibodies raised in the horse can be injected into man to provide a short-lived immunity until injected tetanus toxoid generates a primary antibody response.

LYMPHOKINES

A range of soluble substances with various biological activities is released by lymphocytes (mainly T cells, Table 6.1). The basis of cell-mediated immunity is that lymphokines from a

Table 6.1 Some lymphokines and their functions

Lymphokine	Function
Skin reactive factor	Increases vascular permeability
Lymphotoxin	Cell death
Macrophage inhibition factor	Immobilises macrophages
Chemotactic factors	Chemotactic for macrophages, lymphocytes and eosinophils
Lymphocyte mitogenic factor	Stimulates division of non-sensitised lymphocytes.
Interleukin 2	T lymphocyte proliferation
Fibroblast stimulating factor	Increases collagen production
Interferon	Modulates NK cell activity
Osteoclast-activating factor	Increases bone resorption

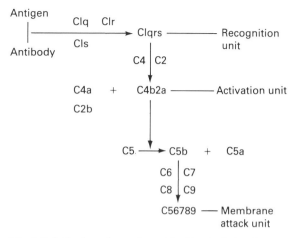

Fig. 6.3 Activation of complement by the classical pathway

few sensitised lymphocytes can recruit other lymphocytes, macrophages and polymorphs in a non-specific manner to produce inflammation. This process takes a few days, hence it is sometimes called *delayed hypersensitivity*.

COMPLEMENT ACTIVATION

The complement system is a series of plasma proteins which, when activated, produces a cascade effect resulting in their deposition on cell membranes, which leads to cell death. In addition, several by-products are formed which have important biological activities.

Classical pathway

The *classical pathway* is activated by antibody–antigen reactions involving IgG or IgM and by proteolytic enzymes such as plasmin or trypsin. Each antibody–antigen complex on cell membranes activates C1 (the *recognition unit*, Fig. 6.3). This generates several *activation units* which appear on the membrane as aggregates of C2 and C4 and which amplify numerous *membrane attack units* consisting of several complement proteins. Each antibody–antigen complex yields multiple membrane attack units. Complement activation produces several results:

1. *Membrane lysis*, produced by C8 and stabilised by the membrane attack unit.

2. *Chemotaxis* of polymorphs, eosinophils and macrophages, induced by C3a, C5a, and C567 complex. (The suffix 'a' denotes an activated by-product.)

3. *Kinin-like activity* (i.e. vascular dilatation and smooth muscle contraction) from C2 activation. In *hereditary angioedema*, most patients have a deficiency of the enzyme required to degrade this activated fragment, and the result is severe oedema which may cause death if the larynx is affected.

4. *Cell death*; C3a is toxic to cells (e.g. fibroblasts).

Alternate pathway

The *alternate pathway* is activated by immunoglobin aggregates, endotoxins, bacterial lipopolysaccharides and proteolytic enzymes. The end result is membrane attack unit formation, but it can take place without antibody-antigen reactions and utilises different enzymes and proteins from the classical pathway in its early stages. Both pathways involve cleavage of C3 to produce C3a, and this can be used clinically to detect complement activation.

IMMUNODEFICIENT STATES

Although numerous causes exist (Table 6.2), primary immunodeficiencies are much rarer than secondary ones.

Table 6.2 Immunodeficient states

Primary immunodeficiencies

  B cells
    Infantile X-linked hypogammaglobulinaemia
    Selective immunoglobulin deficiencies

  T cells
    Congenital thymic aplasia (Di George's syndrome)

  B and T cells
    Severe combined immunodeficiency disease

  Complement deficiencies
    Hereditary angioedema

  Deficiencies of phagocytosis
    Agranulocytosis
    Cyclical neutropenia
    Juvenile periodontitis

Secondary immunodeficiencies

  Drugs
    Immunosuppressants
    Cytotoxics
    Steroids

  Myeloproliferative diseases
    Leukaemia
    Lymphoma
    Myeloma

  Metabolic diseases
    Malnutrition
    Uraemia
    Diabetes mellitus
    Iron deficiency anaemia

  Infections
    Acquired immune deficiency syndrome

Primary immunodeficiencies

In *infantile X-linked hypogammaglobulinaemia*, there is an inherited B cell differentiation defect producing very low immunoglobulin levels; recurrent bacterial infections develop when maternal antibody levels fall at about 6 months of age.

Selective immunoglobulin deficiencies are characterised by a failure to produce one or more immunoglobulin class; IgA is the commonest, and recurrent oral ulceration is frequently seen.

In *congenital thymic aplasia*, there is failure of pharyngeal pouch development producing thymic and parathyroid defects which cause recurrent infections and hypocalcaemic tetany.

Both *T and B cell* deficiencies exist in *severe combined immunodeficiency disease*, another inherited condition; death from infections often occurs within the first year of life.

Secondary immunodeficiencies

These include myeloproliferative and blood diseases (Chapter 20).

Acquired immune deficiency syndrome (AIDS) is caused by the human immunodeficiency virus (HIV). It usually affects male homosexuals, although heterosexuals, particularly intravenous drug addicts and patients (often haemophiliacs) receiving blood or blood products from infected donors, are also at risk. Numerous immunological abnormalities have been described in T, B and NK cells, including alterations in T helper: suppressor cell ratios and abnormal chemotaxis and phagocytosis. A persistent generalised lymphadenopathy may precede AIDS in some patients, and opportunistic infections by parasites, fungi and viruses are common (e.g. *Pneumocystis carinii* pneumonia, candidosis and toxoplasmosis). The head and neck may be the site of recurrent oral infections or cervical lymphadenopathy: many patients develop oral Kaposi's sarcoma, an unusual vascular neoplasm so rarely seen in the mouth that its occurrence in a young male is highly suggestive of AIDS. Prognosis is poor, most patients dying from overwhelming infections or Kaposi's sarcoma.

HYPERSENSITIVITY REACTIONS

These are immunological reactions damaging to tissues, and four types are recognised.

Type I (anaphylaxis). Here, IgE is produced in reaction to antigen. Mast cells bind IgE to their surface, and when the antigen is re-introduced it binds to the IgE to produce mast cell degranulation. This releases histamine and serotonin, causing oedema (due to vascular dilatation and increased permeability) and impaired breathing (due to bronchiolar smooth muscle constriction). This reaction may be caused by allergies to drugs (e.g. penicillin) or food, and is the basis of asthma (allergy to house mites) and hayfever (allergy to pollens). Reasons for the initial production of IgE antibodies are unknown.

Type II (cytotoxic antibody). This involves cell damage caused by antibodies against cell surface molecules and mediated by complement activation or ADCC. Examples include haemolysis following incompatible blood transfusion, haemolytic anaemia and drug-induced thrombocytopaenic purpura.

Type III (immune complex disease). This results from deposition of antigen and antibodies bound together as complexes. In tissues, this produces the *Arthus reaction*, whereas circulating complexes can cause *serum sickness*. In either case, there is inflammation in vessel walls (vasculitis), with necrosis, thrombosis and haemorrhage. Complexes deposited in vessel walls or trapped in basement membranes (e.g. glomerular) activate complement, the chemotactic by-products of which attract polymorphs to the site, where they release lysosomal enzymes to produce vessel and tissue damage. Complement C3b bound to complexes may be responsible for their binding to cells expressing C3b receptors (e.g. endothelial cells and platelets; the latter release vasoactive amines contributing to vasodilatation and clump together to form a thrombus). Examples include some glomerulonephritis (Chapter 18), some drug reactions, lupus erythematosus (Chapter 25) and rheumatoid arthritis.

Type IV (delayed hypersensitivity). Whereas types I to III involve antibody reactions, type IV involves T lymphocytes and lymphokines. It is the basis of the Mantoux test in which tuberculoprotein is injected into the skin; if immunity to tuberculosis already exists, inflammation develops at the injection site after an initial delay. Skin rashes caused by metals and other haptens (contact dermatitis) are mediated by type IV hypersensitivity, the Langerhans' cells of the skin playing an important role in trapping and processing the antigens.

HLA (HUMAN LEUCOCYTE ANTIGEN) SYSTEM

This is a series of inherited antigens, coded on chromosome 6 and expressed on all nucleated cell surfaces (hence its absence from red blood cells; leucocytes were the first cells on which they were found). Cells express one antigen from each parent for each of the four loci (A,B,C,D). As many different antigens exist for each locus, the chance of finding two individuals with identical antigens is remote.

Functions. The HLA system has three main functions:

1. It is the basis of graft rejection. Tissue typing identifies the surface antigens and is used to choose the most suitable donor whose antigens match best those of the recipient; failure to do so leads to rapid rejection (see below).

2. It helps to control the immune system through *immune response (Ir) genes* which can influence antibody production. For example, resistance to dental caries correlates with HLA-D6 antigen which allows stimulation of T helper cells by low (as opposed to high) doses of oral streptococcal antigens.

3. It influences susceptibility to and progression of some diseases. There are many examples of patients with a particular disease sharing a common HLA antigen—in ankylosing spondylitis, 90% express B27, compared with 5% of the normal population; psoriasis is more common in people with HLA-Cw6, and if B27 is also present, there is an increased risk of psoriatic arthritis; AIDS patients have a greater frequency of HLA-DR5; in coeliac disease and dermatitis herpetiformis (a vesicular skin eruption secondary to small intestinal villous atrophy) HLA-B8 is more common than in normal patients. Reasons why there should be genetic predispositions to disease are unknown; several hypotheses have been considered, including specific disease genes lying alongside those for HLA antigens and inherited with them, influence of Ir genes and HLA antigens acting as receptors for pathogenic organisms.

AUTOIMMUNE DISEASES

Here, the immune system reacts against body tissues. Reasons for this are unknown, but possible explanations include modification of cell surface molecules by drugs (e.g. methyldopa-associated haemolytic anaemia), cross-reaction with foreign antigens (e.g. between heart and streptococcal antigens in rheumatic fever) and impaired immune system homeostasis.

Some autoimmune diseases involve only single organs (e.g. thyrotoxicosis and Addison's disease), whilst others affect numerous sites (e.g. systemic lupus erythematosus and rheumatoid arthritis). In thyrotoxicosis, an antibody (long-acting thyroid stimulator) is produced against thyroid cell surfaces; it combines with TSH receptors, thus activating the adenyl cyclase system to stimulate thyroid hormone production. In rheumatoid arthritis, rheumatoid factor (an IgM) is produced against the body's IgG.

Autoimmune diseases frequently occur in middle-aged women, and several may co-exist (e.g. megaloblastic anaemia and autoimmune thyroiditis). Autoantibodies are not uncommon in the general population (e.g. many have antibodies against epidermal cell cytoplasm), but these rarely lead to overt disease.

GRAFT REACTIONS

Autografts can be used to correct bone defects, to by-pass blocked coronary arteries or to repair skin burns. Because the body's own tissues are used, there is no graft rejection.

Homografts in clinical practice include corneal transplantation, but as the cornea is an immuno-privileged site lacking Langerhans cells and is avascular, rejection does not develop, despite unmatched HLA antigens of donor and recipient. On the other hand, bone marrow, heart or kidney transplants will be rejected unless preventive steps are taken. Syngeneic homografts, being HLA identical, are not rejected.

Heterografts have no clinical use, but human pathological material (e.g. tumours) can be grafted under the skin of the nude mouse, a mutant species that is T cell deficient; rejection does not occur, thus allowing biological behaviour to be studied.

Results. The importance of the HLA system in grafting is seen when skin grafted between identical twins survives for 120 days, whereas in non-identical twins rejection takes place by 12 days. As grafting between identical twins is subject to rejection, albeit slowly, other non-HLA antigens must also be involved. Similarly, 90% of grafted kidneys are intact after 1 year in HLA-matched siblings, compared with 60% in non-HLA-matched siblings and 50% if the non-matched donor and host are not related. To obtain the best results, it is necessary to ensure that donor and recipient are of the same blood group and are matched as closely as possible for HLA antigens. To induce tolerance during which time the body is 'tricked' into accepting the graft as its own tissue, drugs (e.g. steroids and azathioprine) are used to immunosuppress the patient; unfortunately, they compromise the immune system and decrease resistance to infection. Tolerance is also a feature of young animals whose immune systems have not fully developed. Injecting newborn mice with cells from a different strain will permit successful allogeneic homografting to the treated mouse during adulthood.

Rejection. Three stages exist:

1. *Hyperacute rejection* ocurs within minutes and is due to ABO incompatibility or prior recipient sensitisation to donor antigens. Red cell sludging, thrombosis and necrosis ensue and are antibody mediated.
2. *Acute rejection* develops within 1–2 weeks, and is due mainly to T cell activation.
3. *Late (chronic) rejection* is mainly B cell mediated, and develops a considerable time after grafting. It is due to a gradual escape of antigens from immunosuppression, and antibodies are produced to endothelial cells within the graft.

Graft versus Host (GvH) disease. In GvH disease, host tissues tolerate the graft, but immunocompetent cells in the graft attack 'foreign' recipient antigens. GvH disease may complicate bone marrow transplantation in leukaemic patients given whole body irradiation to kill abnormal and immunocompetent recipient cells. Poor HLA matching increases the likelihood of a GvH reaction. Clinically, there may be skin eruptions, jaundice, infection and even death.

DENTAL ASPECTS

Numerous lymphoid aggregates are present in the mouth, including larger lymph nodes such as Waldeyer's ring and the many small lymphoid structures embedded in oral mucosa. Saliva contains IgA as well as serum antibodies which have emerged from the gingiva via crevicular fluid.

Dental caries. In the first few months of life, infants obtain antibodies to bacterial plaque by natural passive immunisation from their mothers' milk, but these disappear before the first tooth erupts at six months of age. Accordingly, the infant has few antibodies to its own plaque bacteria, and a critical period exists between removal of maternal antibodies, colonisation of newly erupted teeth by plaque bacteria and development of the child's own immunity. Plaque can be attacked by antibodies produced in gingiva and transported by crevicular fluid; the latter can also carry polymorphs into the saliva. Plaque contains many substances capable of both stimulating and inhibiting local immune responses (e.g. lipopolysaccharides, dextrans and levans). *Streptococcus mutans* is probably the most important cariogenic bacterium, and attempts to raise vaccines against it are in progress. Patients vary in their susceptibility to dental caries and their immune responses to plaque bacteria and extracts; some 3% are caries resistant, and show high serum antibody titres, a greater tendency for T cells to proliferate on stimulation with streptococcal antigen and an efficient HLA-associated T helper cell activity.

Periodontal disease. Periodontal tissue destruction is due to the long term presence of plaque bacteria on cervical margins of teeth causing chronic inflammation. In gingivitis, the infiltrating lymphocytes are mainly T cells, and the disease is stable, with little continued destruction; however, in advanced periodontitis with bone loss, B cells predominate and are not under the same degree of negative feedback as the earlier T cells. Reasons for this T to B shift are unknown but probably important. Evidence implicating immunological reactions in periodontitis comes from several sources: immunodeficient or immunosuppressed patients have less gingivitis, and patients taking levamisole (a T cell stimulator) develop more gingivitis; in juvenile periodontitis, where rapid bone loss is seen in young patients, polymorph chemotaxis is defective, stimulation of lymphocyte proliferation by plaque is decreased and immunoglobulin levels are altered. Initial tissue damage is due to complement activation by either pathway causing vasodilatation and polymorph chemotaxis. Lymphokines from T cells and lysosomal enzymes from polymorphs and macrophages cause collagen loss; cytotoxic T cells and ADCC also contribute to tissue damage. Prostaglandin release, osteoclast-activating factor (from B cells) and bacterial endotoxin produce bone loss.

Oral infections. In general, patients with a B cell immunodeficiency have recurrent bacterial infections; T cell immunodeficiency predisposes to recurrent viral and fungal infections (e.g. herpes simplex and *Candida*). Patients with *recurrent herpes simplex* may have interferon and macrophage inhibition factor deficiencies. In chronic mucocutaneous *candidosis*, patients have antibodies against candicidal factors in serum; systemic candidosis may be associated with abnormal phagocytic cell chemotaxis and defective lysosomal enzyme and T cell functions.

7

Miscellaneous tissue deposits

Amyloidosis
Heterotopic calcification
Gout
Pigmentation
Exogenous
Endogenous
Dental aspects

AMYLOIDOSIS

Amyloidosis is a disorder characterised by extra-cellular tissue deposits of an abnormal protein, amyloid.

Staining characteristics. Amyloid identification is based almost entirely on its staining properties. Macroscopically, *iodine solution* produces a mahogany-brown colour; histologically, *Congo red* imparts a brick-red colour which, under polarized light, shows green birefringence.

Physical and chemical characteristics. Approximately 90% of amyloid protein consists of unbranching fibrils aggregated into β-pleated sheets; the remainder is a non-fibrillar glycoprotein *amyloid P component* (AP). Two major amyloid proteins are recognised: *amyloid light chain* (AL), derived from plasma cells and containing immunoglobulin light chains, and a unique non-immunoglobulin protein of uncertain origin but probably derived from a larger serum precursor, *amyloid associated* (AA). Although these variants form the basis of some modern classifications, traditional classifications are still more widely used, and will be discussed here.

Forms. There are two major (primary and secondary) and three much less common types.

Primary (immunocyte-derived) amyloidosis occurs without any obvious cause, and is seen mainly in the heart, gastrointestinal tract and tongue (which can be considerably enlarged—macroglossia). Amyloidosis associated with multiple myeloma (Chapter 20) has a similar distribution.

Secondary (reactive systemic) amyloidosis is associated with chronic inflammatory conditions such as rheumatoid arthritis, chronic osteomyelitis, bronchiectasis, tuberculosis and Crohn's disease. It is seen mainly in spleen, liver and kidneys (where glomerular deposits can produce the nephrotic syndrome—Chapter 18); it may be laid down in the gingiva, which can be biopsied for diagnostic purposes.

Hereditary amyloidosis is rare; the commonest example is *familial Mediterranean fever*, an autosomal recessive condition accompanied by inflammation of serosal surfaces including peritoneum, pleura and synovial membranes.

Localised amyloidosis is limited to a single organ or tissue, most commonly lung, larynx and tongue; it can also occur in tissues and tumours of the APUD system (Chapter 10).

Senile amyloidosis is characterised by small deposits in the brain and heart; occasionally the cardiac involvement may be marked, causing heart failure.

HETEROTOPIC CALCIFICATION

Heterotopic calcification, (i.e. abnormal calcium deposition) occurs in tissues not normally associated with mineralisation.

In *dystrophic calcification*, plasma calcium and phosphate levels are normal, and calcium salts are deposited in degenerate and necrotic tissues. *Caseous material* in tuberculous lesions commonly calcifies, as seen in healed pulmonary Ghon foci and tuberculous lymphadenitis in the neck or intestinal mesentery. *Dead parasites*, including *Trichinella spiralis*, schistosome ova and hydatid cysts, often calcify, as may long-standing venous or arterial *thrombi* and established *haematomas*. Other sites include *mature granulation tissue, scar tissue, atheromatous plaques, fibrous epulis, dental pulp* (where pulp stones can form), *traumatic fat necrosis* and certain *tumours* (e.g. breast carcinomas, where it can be detected by mammography).

In *metastatic calcification*, plasma calcium levels are raised (hypercalcaemia). This occurs with hyperparathyroidism (Chapter 19), excessive intestinal calcium absorption in hypervitaminosis D and osteolytic metastatic tumour deposits (Chapter 22). The most common site is around renal tubules and in the renal pelvis (producing nephrocalcinosis and calculi respectively—Chapter 18); other sites include lungs, stomach, blood vessels and cornea.

GOUT

Gout is an uncommon, often familial disease occurring predominantly in males over 50 years of age and is characterised by deposition of sodium biurate crystals in many sites, particularly peri-articular tissues. There are increased serum uric acid levels due to either increased uric acid synthesis (as in *primary gout*, which is probably an inborn error of metabolism) or increased nucleoprotein breakdown (*secondary gout*, e.g. in patients with leukaemia and polycythaemia, especially following cytotoxic drug treatment).

In *acute gout*, the joint involved is swollen, red and extremely painful; peri-articular tissues are distended with crystalline deposits, and urate crystals may be expressed through the overlying skin.

In *chronic gout*, hard, white localised nodules (*tophi*) are found around joints, particularly the first metatarso-phalangeal joint, and elsewhere, often in ear cartilages, subcutaneous tissues, bursae and kidneys.

PIGMENTATION

Pigments, some of which are normal cellular constituents, may, under abnormal conditions, accumulate in cells and tissues.

Exogenous

Exogenous pigments are absorbed from the gut, inhaled or injected.

Silver can produce brownish grey granules giving a dusky appearance to the skin.

Lead and bismuth can cause characteristic 'blue lines' on gingivae.

Inhaled *carbon particles* produce black pigmentation of the lungs (anthracosis); in coal miners, this can result in serious lung disease (Chapter 14). A rust-like discolouration (*siderosis*) is seen in lungs following long-term exposure to *iron-ore particles*.

In *tattooing*, coarse pigment particles are injected into the skin. Dental amalgam fragments implanted into oral soft tissues during operative procedures elicit various reactions including giant cell formation; clinically, bluish-brown pigmentation results (*amalgam tattoo*).

Endogenous

Endogenous pigments are mainly derived from melanin or haemoglobin.

Melanin is brown-black pigment formed in melanocytes when tyrosinase catalyses tryrosine oxidation to dihydroxyphenylalanine (DOPA). Increased melanin pigmentation occurs during exposure to *sunlight, pregnancy* and in *Addison's disease* (Chapter 19); striking oral mucosal pigmentation occurs with the Peutz–Jeghers syndrome (Chapter 16); *melanosis coli* is brownish pigmentation of colonic mucosa by pigment-containing macrophages. *Leukoderma* (vitiligo) is patchy skin depigmentation due to failure of melanocytes to oxidise DOPA to form pigment. Both benign and malignant melanocyte tumours can produce excess melanin pigment (Chapter 25).

Haemoglobin produces several different pigments:

Haematin, a dark brown pigment, is found with very severe acute red cell destruction (e.g. incompatible blood transfusion reactions and malaria, when it appears in the urine—Blackwater fever).

Haemosiderin presents in two ways: *haemosiderosis* is generalised iron overload in the body, and is secondary to prolonged and excessive oral iron intake, multiple blood transfusions or increased red cell breakdown in haemolytic anaemias;

haemochromatosis is iron overload due to an inherited inborn error of iron metabolism. There is excessive intestinal absorption of iron, with deposition in many organs including *liver* (where cirrhosis may develop), *pancreas* (where Islets of Langerhans are gradually destroyed and diabetes mellitus may develop) and *skin* (which shows bronze pigmentation due mainly to increased melanin deposition but also to occasional subcutaneous haemosiderin-laden macrophages).

Bilirubin is a normal breakdown product of red cells which is removed from plasma by the liver and excreted in bile. Excess red cell breakdown, liver cell disturbances or biliary tract obstruction will cause plasma bilirubin levels to rise, producing *jaundice* (Chapter 17).

Porphyrins, the respiratory pigments of red cells, are normally present in only very small quantities in plasma and urine. In *porphyria*, inborn errors of metabolism produce considerably elevated plasma and urine porphyrin levels; the urine is dark red in colour, photosensitivity is common and there may be red-brown discoloration of teeth and bones.

Lipofuscin, a yellow-brown pigment with a high lipid content, is found in elderly individuals and is considered a 'wear-and-tear' pigment. It is seen in myocardial fibres (producing brown atrophy of the heart) and elsewhere, particularly liver and nerve cells, odontogenic cysts of the jaw and salivary gland neoplasms.

DENTAL ASPECTS

Some have already been mentioned above.

Pigmentation of teeth has two major causes:

1. Change in structure or thickness during formation. Poorly formed enamel or dentine (as in amelogenesis or dentinogenesis imperfecta) produces brown teeth. Excess *fluoride* causes chalky white/brown enamel discoloration. In *internal resorption* of erupted teeth, osteoclast-like cells in the pulp remove dentine irregularly, producing *pink spots* where dentine is thinned over vascular pulp tissue; eventually, dentine and enamel may perforate.

2. Uptake of colouring agents. These include *tetracyclines* (yellow/brown staining), porphyrins in *porphyria* (red, especially in UV light) and *haemolytic disease of the newborn* (green discoloration by bilirubin) during tooth formation. After tooth eruption, *pulp necrosis* causes teeth to blacken, pigments from *plaque* can cause orange/green staining, *iron* solutions can blacken enamel and *tobacco* produces surface brown staining.

8

Circulatory disturbances

Introduction
Congestion
Oedema
Causes
Haemorrhage
Causes
Shock

Causes and types
Pathological changes
Thrombosis
Causes
Types
Results
Embolism

Types
Ischaemia
Causes
Effects
Infarction
Results

INTRODUCTION

Cell and tissue functions depend on a normal fluid environment and an adequate blood supply; inbalances can result in conditions discussed in this chapter.

CONGESTION

Hyperaemia and Congestion describe an increased volume of blood in affected tissues or organs.

Hyperaemia. This is an active process; sympathetic—neurogenic mechanisms cause arteriolar dilatation, and local redness is produced (e.g. in acute inflammation).

Congestion. This causes bluish colouration due to the accumulation of stagnant blood containing deoxygenated haemoglobin. It follows obstruction of venous return, and is commonly seen in lungs, liver and spleen.

Pulmonary congestion is encountered in left ventricular failure and mitral stenosis (Chapter 13); breakdown and phagocytosis of intra-alveolar red cell debris eventually lead to the accumulation of haemosiderin-laden macrophages (heart-failure cells).

Chronic passive congestion of the liver usually results from right heart failure; red cells accumulate in sinusoids around central veins, producing a contrast with the surrounding paler normal areas to create an appearance referred to as 'nutmeg liver.'

Congestion of the spleen produces enlargement (splenomegaly), focal haemorrhages and, eventually, fibrous scars.

OEDEMA

Oedema is the accumulation of excess fluid in intercellular (interstitial) tissue spaces. In the peritoneal cavity, it is *ascites*; in the pleural cavity, it is a *pleural effusion* (or *hydrothorax*); in the pericardial sac, it is a *pericardial effusion*.

Normal intercellular fluid balance is maintained by two main factors: *hydrostatic pressure* forces fluid from the circulation into intercellular spaces, whilst intravascular *colloid osmotic (oncotic) pressure* attracts it back. In the systemic circulation, capillary hydrostatic pressure at the arterial end is 32–35 mmHg and 12–15 mmHg at the venous end. Plasma colloid osmotic pressure, exerted mainly by albumin, is 20–25 mmHg. Normally, therefore, fluid escapes from the arteriolar end and returns at the venous end; any excess fluid is removed by lymphatics.

Causes

Causes are local or general.

Local

Acute inflammatory oedema, the result of increased capillary permeability, is an *exudate*, rich in protein (Chapter 3); non-inflammatory oedema, low in protein, is a *transudate*.

Hypersensitivity (allergic) oedema is also due to increased vascular permeability (e.g. angioneurotic oedema, Chapter 6).

Venous obstruction (e.g. by thrombus) can produce local oedema by increasing the hydrostatic pressure at the venous end of the capillary network.

Lymphatic oedema results from obstruction of lymph vessels by tumour cells or by traumatic, inflammatory or surgical injuries. A striking example is *filariasis*, where parasitic obstruction causes massive leg oedema (*elephantiasis*).

General

Increased hydrostatic pressure occurs in right ventricular failure (Chapter 13). Oedema distribution is influenced by gravity; thus, in ambulant individuals, ankle oedema is produced, whereas in recumbent patients the oedema appears in the sacral region.

Reduced colloid osmotic pressure reflects hypoalbuminaemia, and usually results from either inadequate synthesis or increased loss; the former is most commonly associated with diffuse liver disease, particularly cirrhosis (Chapter 17): the latter is seen in the nephrotic syndrome (Chapter 18) and rarely with protein-losing intestinal diseases.

HAEMORRHAGE

Haemorrhage is bleeding from ruptured or damaged blood vessels. Haemorrhage into tissues produces a *haematoma*, commonly referred to as a *bruise*. Bleeding into cavities causes *haemothorax*, *haemopericardium* or *haemoperitoneum*. Small haemorrhages into skin and mucous membranes are sometimes termed *petechial* (pin-point) or *purpuric* (up to 1 cm).

Causes

Causes include *trauma* (often involving large vessels), *primary blood vessel disorders* (e.g. atherosclerosis and hypertension—Chapter 12), *damage to normal blood vessels* (e.g. erosion by tumours) and *haemorrhagic diseases* (Chapter 20).

SHOCK

Shock refers to the haemodynamic changes following inadequate tissue perfusion; the effects are produced by hypoxia and accumulation of metabolites.

Causes and types

Cardiogenic shock results from a sudden fall in cardiac output as following myocardial infarction or, much less commonly, open heart surgery, severe myocarditis (Chapter 13) or massive pulmonary embolism (below).

Hypovolaemic shock is produced by a rapid reduction in blood volume. The commonest cause is severe haemorrhage (e.g. trauma, as in road traffic accidents); other causes include extensive burns (with marked transudation and exudation of fluid) and dehydration.

Septic shock is due to bacteraemia or septicaemia by organisms which liberate endotoxins (e.g. gram-negative bacteria such as *E. coli*, *Proteus* or *Pseudomonas* species). Toxins produce arteriolar vasodilatation and pooling of blood which thus reduces the effective circulating volume. Activation of platelets and clotting sequences can induce *disseminated intravascular coagulation* as a complication.

Pathological changes

Pathological changes include cell necrosis, tissue haemorrhages and venous microthrombi. The haemorrhage reflects increased fibrinolysis, thrombocytopenia and hypofibrinogenaemia (Chapter 20). Organ effects include heart failure, intraseptal oedema and plasma protein exudation into alveolar spaces in lungs, acute renal tubular necrosis (causing renal failure) and 'stress ulcers' in stomach and duodenum.

THROMBOSIS

Thrombosis is the formation of a solid mass (*thrombus*) from blood constituents within blood vessels or the heart during life. A *blood clot* is formed when fibrinogen is converted into fibrin by *coagulation* (*clotting*), and this can occur after death.

Causes

Three major factors predispose to thrombosis:

1. *Endothelial injury*; this is seen on ulcerated atheromatous plaques and diseased heart valves, and with arteritis and hypertension (Chapter 12). Platelets adhere to the damaged surface, release thromboplastins and activate coagulation to produce thrombosis.

2. *Alterations of blood flow*, particularly slowing and turbulence. *Slowing* allows platelets to come into contact with the endothelium, thus encouraging aggregation and thrombus formation; such thrombi are common in deep leg veins following bed rest, when reduced muscular activity promotes blood stasis. *Turbulence* is seen over partially obstructive lesions such as atheromatous plaques.

3. *Alteration of blood constituents* producing hypercoagulability. This is seen in such conditions as extensive burns, severe trauma and shock. Certain malignant tumours (e.g. carcinoma of the pancreas) are associated with a predisposition to thrombosis; cancer cells are thought to produce procoagulative factors which may increase platelet activation, raise clotting factor or fibrinogen levels or decrease fibrinolytic activity.

Types

Mural thrombi are found in heart chambers and aorta; thrombi on diseased cardiac valves are referred to as vegetations (Chapter 13).

Occlusive thrombi produce luminal obstruction, and are seen in small arteries (e.g. coronary and cerebral arterial branches).

Venous thrombi (phlebothrombosis) occur in deep leg and superficial varicose veins. Thrombosis within skull venous sinuses may follow severe facial and maxillary acute infections.

Results

Thrombus may occlude a vessel and cause *ischaemia* or *infarction* (see below). Part of a thrombus may dislodge into the blood stream to become an *embolus* (see below). Later, thrombi may be dissolved by *fibrinolysis*, or may undergo *organisation* and *recanalisation* to restore some blood flow.

EMBOLISM

An *embolus* is an abnormal, undissolved solid, liquid or gaseous mass carried by the blood stream; this process, together with its subsequent impaction in vessels, is termed *embolism*.

Types

Thrombotic emboli are the commonest (approximately 95%), and can be arterial or venous.

Arterial or *systemic* emboli usually arise from mural thrombi in the left ventricle following myocardial infarction; less commonly, they may be from the left atrium in atrial fibrillation, aortic atheromatous plaques and aneurysms, or vegetations on diseased heart valve cusps and valve prostheses. They can lodge anywhere in the arterial system, and invariably cause infarction (see below).

Venous emboli are exemplified by *pulmonary embolism*. They invariably originate from deep veins of the legs; following dislodgement, they pass through the right atrium and ventricle to enter the pulmonary circulation. Large emboli can lodge at the pulmonary artery bifurcation, forming *saddle emboli*. More commonly, they occlude major pulmonary vessels or travel to the periphery to occlude smaller arteries. Massive pulmonary embolism will cause sudden death; smaller emboli will produce pulmonary infarction or local intra-pulmonary haemorrhage. Very rarely, an embolus may enter the right side of the heart and pass through an interatrial or interventricular septal defect into the systemic circulation—*paradoxical embolism*.

Fat embolism syndrome is characterised by progressive breathlessness, confusion and sometimes renal failure, and develops 24–72 hours after severe compression of adipose tissue or bone fractures. Fat droplets enter ruptured blood vessels at the site of trauma, and produce embolic occlusion of pulmonary, cerebral and renal vasculature.

Air embolism can occur when air enters large veins following lung, chest or neck injuries. Many small bubbles can coalesce to form large gaseous masses which block pulmonary or cerebral vessels and which may cause sudden death. More than 100 ml is normally required to produce clinical effects; smaller quantities usually dissolve in the plasma. *Caisson disease* occurs when a deep sea diver is brought too rapidly to surface atmospheric pressure. Nitrogen, which under high pressure is dissolved in the plasma, forms numerous small gas emboli on decompression; these emboli obstruct vessels throughout the body, and produce characteristic muscle and joint pains—the *'bends'*.

Amniotic fluid embolism can occur in prolonged labour or traumatic delivery, and is demonstrated by desquamated squamous cells in maternal pulmonary vessels. Typically, it produces cardiovascular shock and respiratory distress, and is thought to be due to anaphylaxis and disseminated intravascular coagulation following entry of amniotic thromboplastins into the maternal circulation.

Malignant tumour cells and fragments from *atheromatous plaques* may embolise.

ISCHAEMIA

Ischaemia indicates inadequate blood supply to an area of tissue.

Causes

The most important and commonest cause is *arterial obstruction* by thrombosis, embolism or progressive atherosclerosis (e.g. coronary, cerebral and renal arteries); *venous obstruction* can occur in varicose veins and produce ischaemic changes in skin; *small vessel and capillary obstruction* is seen in disseminated intravascular coagulation, fat embolism and vasculitis.

Effects

Effects depend upon the adequacy of collateral blood supply; good collaterals will produce little or no effect, whereas poor anastomoses will often result in functional disturbances or even cell death (infarction, below). In the heart, ischaemia causes chest pain (angina); in lower limbs, it produces intermittent claudication (pain in calf muscles during exercise).

INFARCTION

An *infarct* is a localised area of ischaemic necrosis due to sudden decrease in arterial supply or obstruction to venous drainage; macroscopically, it is usually white or red.

White (pale or anaemic) infarcts follow arterial occlusion in solid organs with no significant collateral circulation (e.g. heart, spleen and kidneys).

Red (haemorrhagic) infarcts usually follow venous occlusion or occur in tissues with reasonable collateral or double circulations (e.g. intestines and lungs). The colour reflects the amount of blood which accumulates in the parenchyma during infarction.

Septic infarcts are due to emboli containing pyogenic bacteria (e.g. from infected vegetations on diseased heart valves).

Results

Infarcts, particularly in lungs, kidneys and spleen, are often wedge shaped, with the base at the periphery of the organ and the apex adjacent to the occluded vessel. Infarction everywhere except in the brain produces *coagulative necrosis*; this stimulates an acute inflammatory cell response followed by organisation and, ultimately, fibrous scar formation. In the brain, infarction produces *colliquative necrosis* followed by glial cell proliferation and eventually gliosis. In septic infarcts, abscesses may develop.

9

Disorders of cell growth and development

Aplasia
Hypoplasia
Atrophy
Hypertrophy
Hyperplasia
Hamartomas

Heterotopia
Developmental cysts
Metaplasia
Dysplasia
Atypia
Neoplasia

APLASIA

Aplasia (*agenesis*) is the complete failure of development of a tissue or organ. It is most commonly seen in paired organs such as kidneys and adrenals, when one or both may be involved, and can affect the teeth—for example, missing third molars or even, in severe inherited forms, absence of an entire dentition.

HYPOPLASIA

Hypoplasia is the inability or failure of an organ to develop to its normal mature size. Such rudimentary organs lack the full complement of cells, resulting in reduced functional activity. In enamel hypoplasia, enamel matrix secretion is reduced; in its mild form, pitting results, but when severe (as in amelogenesis imperfecta), there is flaking and loss of abnormal enamel from every tooth.

ATROPHY

Atrophy is an *acquired* reduction in organ or tissue mass due to a decrease in number and size of its constituent cells (cf. hypoplasia).

Physiological atrophy

Physiological atrophy is seen in many structures during fetal development, including notochord, thyroglossal duct and branchial clefts; during infancy, it occurs in the thymus and adrenal cortex. A dramatic example is the uterine wall after childbirth. *Senile atrophy* involves many tissues; it represents physiological change associated with ageing and decreased endocrine organ activity.

Pathological atrophy

Pathological atrophy may be general or local.

General atrophy is associated with starvation from famine, chronic illnesses such as tuberculosis, malabsorption syndrome (Chapter 16) and malignant disease (*cachexia*).

Local atrophy has several forms. *Disuse atrophy* is most commonly seen in voluntary muscles following immobilisation for bone fractures. Joint diseases which limit movement by pain or deformity (e.g. rheumatoid arthritis) and loss of motor nerve supply (e.g. following trauma or poliomyelitis) also produce muscle atrophy. Accumulation of secretions behind duct obstruction (e.g. by calculi) will produce *pressure atrophy* in organs such as salivary glands, pancreas and kidneys. *Endocrine gland atrophy* occurs in the absence of trophic pituitary hormones (e.g. adrenocorticotrophic hormone, ACTH, and thyroid-stimulating hormone, TSH) or can be iatrogenic as seen in the adrenal cortex in long term steroid administration.

HYPERTROPHY

Hypertrophy is the increase in organ or tissue mass due to an increase in *size* of its constituent cells.

Physiological hypertrophy

Physiological hypertrophy is seen in the uterus during pregnancy and in skeletal muscles in trained athletes.

Pathological hypertrophy

Pathological hypertrophy is adaptive or compensatory.

Adaptive hypertrophy occurs in hollow muscular organs whenever outflow disturbances produce increased mechanical resistance. This is seen in the heart in systemic hypertension and valvular diseases; smooth muscle hypertrophy develops in the bladder following progressive prostatic enlargement and in the stomach in pyloric stenosis.

Compensatory hypertrophy is seen in paired organs such as kidneys and adrenals, and occurs when one organ is damaged or removed. Under these circumstances, there is usually also an associated element of hyperplasia.

Hypertrophy requires healthy tissue as well as an adequate stimulus. In muscular hypertrophy, initial stretching stimulates the increase in size; in compensatory hypertrophy, mechanisms are not fully understood, but in endocrine organs surviving glandular tissue is stimulated by appropriate pituitary hormones.

HYPERPLASIA

Hyperplasia is the increase in organ or tissue mass due to an increase in *number* of its constituent cells. When the causative agent is removed, regression will follow (cf. neoplasia).

Physiological hyperplasia

Physiological hyperplasia, invariably accompanied by hypertrophy, occurs in organs influenced by hormones (e.g. breasts and uterus).

Pathological hyperplasia

Pathological hyperplasia is classically seen in endocrine organs.

Diffuse hyperplasia involves the entire organ, and the resulting increase in hormone secretion produces functional changes. Examples include parathyroid glands in chronic renal failure and thyroid in Graves' disease (Chapter 19).

Focal hyperplasia produces discrete nodules, and occurs in adrenals and parathyroids.

Bone marrow hyperplasia is associated with some anaemias; normal adult marrow is yellowish because of its fat, but with pronounced hyperplasia it appears red as a result of increased haemopoiesis.

Lymphoid hyperplasia, involving lymph nodes and sometimes the spleen, is seen in many chronic infections.

Connective tissue hyperplasia may produce localised overgrowths of fibrous tissue; these are common in the mouth, induced by inflammation (*gingival epulis*), ill-fitting dentures (*denture irritation hyperplasia*), trauma (e.g. a *fibro-epithelial polyp* of buccal mucosa) or epanutin given to control epilepsy (*epanutin hyperplasia*).

Pseudo-epitheliomatous hyperplasia is epithelial thickening associated with chronic inflammation and characterised by greatly elongated rete ridges; sometimes, it can be difficult to distinguish histologically from early squamous cell carcinoma.

HAMARTOMA

Hamartoma is a malformation in which there is an excess of one or more of the constituents normally found in the tissue or organ concerned.

Vascular hamartomas are the commonest.

Capillary haemangiomas, comprising small capillaries, occur mainly in the skin, where they form well-defined lesions often referred to as 'birth marks'; they usually regress spontaneously, but surgical removal may be necessary.

Cavernous haemangiomas, composed of large interconnecting sinus-like vascular spaces, are found on the lips and tongue, and internally in liver and bone; those in the jaw bones may cause excessive haemorrhage on tooth extraction.

Hereditary haemorrhagic telangiectasia, inherited as an autosomal dominant, is characterised by multiple small telangiectatic spots (arteriolar-venular anastomoses) in skin, mucous membranes (e.g. nose) and lungs; such lesions can be a site of bleeding (Chapter 20).

Lymphangioma is a hamartoma of lymphatic

vessels; one type occurs in infancy as a swelling in the neck—a cystic hygroma.

Other hamartomas include abnormalities of developing dental tissues (*odontomes*) where enamel, dentine, cementum and pulp are arranged haphazardly; occasionally, a tooth-like denticle is formed, but frequently an irregular mass is produced.

HETEROTOPIA

Heterotopia is an organ or tissue in an abnormal site. Examples include thyroid tissue at the upper end of the thyroglossal duct (the 'lingual thyroid') and pancreatic tissue in the wall of the stomach or small intestine.

DEVELOPMENTAL CYSTS

Developmental cysts may arise from heterotopic tissue or from persisting vestigial epithelial remnants.

Dermoid cysts, which contain keratin and sebum, are lined by stratified squamous epithelium and may have sebaceous glands, sweat glands or hair follicles in their wall; they usually develop in subcutaneous tissues, but may be found under the tongue (sublingual dermoid).

Branchial cysts arise from persisting cervical sinuses, and are lined by stratified squamous epithelium and lymphoid tissue.

Thyroglossal cysts develop from remnants of the thyroglossal duct following migration of the thyroid from the base of the tongue; such cysts often incorporate thyroid tissue in their walls.

Developmental cysts of the jaws arise either from odontogenic epithelium (odontogenic developmental cysts) or from epithelial remnants trapped in bone during embryogenesis (non-odontogenic developmental, or fissural, cysts). *Odontogenic developmental cysts* include *dentigerous cysts* arising in dental follicles around unerupted teeth; their linings are derived from reduced enamel epithelium surrounding the crown after its morphogenesis is complete. *Fissural cysts* include those developing in the midline of the palate and between upper and lateral incisors and canine teeth (*globulomaxillary cysts*).

METAPLASIA

Metaplasia is the change from one type of tissue to another related but often less specialised type, and most frequently affects epithelium.

Squamous metaplasia is usually initiated by chronic inflammation and prolonged irritation; it is seen in the gallbladder and urinary bladder, particularly when calculi are present, and in the bronchial tree as a result of irritation from smoking. Widespread squamous metaplasia of respiratory and salivary epithelium is associated with vitamin A deficiency.

In chronic bronchitis, pseudostratified ciliated respiratory epithelium can change to simple mucus-secreting columnar type (*mucous metaplasia*).

Connective tissue metaplasia is seen in scar tissue with osteoid and bone production (*osseous metaplasia*).

DYSPLASIA

Dysplasia usually indicates the general disturbance in architecture of an epithelium showing cellular atypia (see below). Unfortunately, the term is occasionally used to denote abnormal tissue development (e.g. renal dysplasia and fibrous dysplasia).

ATYPIA

Atypia refers to the morphological changes of individual epithelial cells which reflect abnormal proliferation and differentiation, and includes nuclear hyperchromatism (increased staining), cellular and/or nuclear pleomorphism (variation in size and shape), abnormal mitoses, premature keratinization and loss of the normal maturation sequence from basal layer to surface. Such appearances may indicate a greater risk of carcinoma developing from the abnormal epithelium (Chapter 10).

NEOPLASIA

Neoplasia, an abnormal proliferation of cells, is the subject of Chapter 10.

10

Neoplasia

Definition   Genetic influences   **Grading and staging of malignant neoplasms**
Stages of carcinogenesis   **Occupation-related neoplasms**   **In vitro characteristics of malignancy**
Target cell population   **Classification**   **Effects**
Causes   Behaviour   Benign tumours
Physical agents   Histogenesis   Malignant tumours
Chemical carcinogens   **Premalignancy**   **Tumour markers**
Viruses   **Spread of malignant neoplasms**

DEFINITION

A *neoplasm* is an abnormal tissue mass or cell population with an ability for progressive and uncontrolled growth. Most produce definite lumps—hence the alternative name *tumour*. Unlike hyperplasia (Chapter 9), it continues to grow in the same excessive manner when the 'stimulus' which caused it is removed.

STAGES OF CARCINOGENESIS

Carcinogenesis has two main stages—*initiation* and *promotion*. Initiation is rapid and irreversible, and requires a relatively small amount of a cancer-causing agent (*carcinogen*); promotion increases the subsequent tumour-producing response. If a single dose of inititator, such as dimethylbenzanthracene (DMBA) is painted on skin and followed up to 1 year later by repeated doses of a promotor, for example 12-0-tetradecanoylphorbol-13-acetate (TPA), papillomas develop after a latent interval. Promotor or initiator alone, or promotor given before initiator, fail to produce neoplasms. In skin, promotors cause epithelial hyperplasia and lead to an expansion of clones of initiated cells. However, promotors are complex, and may act via many biochemical pathways; saccharin, cyclamates and oestrogens may act as promotors in different tissues. Carcinogenesis is a prolonged *multistage process* (see experiment described above). Doubt exists about the number of carcinogenic events required, but it may often be three to five; in mouse skin, these comprise initiation and at least two distinct promotional stages.

Human carcinogenesis also involves a long time scale; the peak incidence of epithelial malignancy in Hiroshima and Nagasaki atom bomb survivors occurred 20 years later, fibrosarcomas may develop decades after irradiation and mesothelioma often appears 20 years after asbestos exposure.

TARGET CELL POPULATION

A consequence of the long time scale is seen in renewing cell populations (e.g. bone marrow and surface epithelia), where most initiated cells will have differentiated into mature end cells before subsequent carcinogenic events occur. The more steps required for malignant transformation, the greater is the probability that important target cells must have been present throughout the entire process and be capable of long term proliferation. The only cells likely to fulfil these requirements are the *stem cells* which comprise only a small proportion of basal cells in skin and oral mucosa and are the least mature cells in bone marrow. They have the greatest division potential and give rise to the remaining proliferating cells which are ultimately destined to differentiate. In some tissues (e.g. intestinal crypts and filiform tongue papillae) they are located deeply so that their daughter cells migrate from stem cell zones along basement membranes towards the surface.

CAUSES

Physical agents

Physical agents include ionising and ultraviolet radiation. The association between neoplasia and ionising radiation was noted soon after X-rays were discovered, when workers were found to have an increased incidence of skin cancer and leukaemia. Ultraviolet radiation can promote skin cancers; this association is dramatically seen in fair-skinned people exposed to prolonged sunshine as in parts of Australia. Radiation damages DNA, alters cellular proteins and inactivates enzymes (Chapter 11).

Chemical carcinogens

Chemical carcinogens are synthetic or natural; many are *precarcinogens*, requiring enzymatic activation in the body to produce the active or ultimate carcinogen.

Synthetic

Polycyclic hydrocarbons are derived from the anthracene nucleus, and include benzanthracene and benzpyrene. The major source is burning fossil fuels (e.g. heating systems, industrial plants, internal combustion and aircraft engines); they are also found in foods cooked in fat and oil or smoked. Naturally occurring compounds (e.g. bile salts and cholesterol) may be converted, by intestinal bacteria, to polycyclic hydrocarbons.

Aromatic amines are by-products of tar formation. One, naphthylamine, was used in aniline dye and rubber industries and was responsible for a marked increase in bladder cancer among workers. The ultimate carcinogen, 2-amino-1-phenol, is produced in the liver, inactivated by conjugation with glucuronic acid and excreted in the urine; however, in susceptible subjects, bladder epithelium can secrete β glucuronidase, which releases active carcinogen.

Amino-azo dyes (e.g. scarlet red and butter yellow) were formerly used for food colouring.

Natural

Natural chemical carcinogens are usually food contaminants.

Mycotoxins are produced by fungi. Aflatoxin is from the common mould *Aspergillus flavus*, and is found on improperly stored grains and peanuts; it causes liver cancer in animals, and may contribute to human liver cancer in certain parts of Africa.

Nitrosamines, potent carcinogens, are present in minute amounts in cigarette smoke, alcoholic beverages and certain foods, and they are also formed, in the stomach, from nitrate preservative present in tinned foods; in addition, they may be manufactured from harmless precursors by intestinal bacteria.

Heavy metals, such as chromium and beryllium, can induce cancer either by emitting ionising radiation or by reacting with nucleic acid phosphate groups in DNA.

Asbestos, when inhaled, is related to pleural (mesothelioma) and bronchial neoplasia.

Viruses

Viruses are associated with several animal tumours (e.g. fowl and feline leukaemia, fowl sarcoma, rabbit skin papilloma and mouse mammary carcinoma); in humans, they have been implicated, but as yet conclusive evidence has not been fully established.

RNA tumour viruses (*oncornaviruses*) contain the enzyme reverse transcriptase (an RNA-directed DNA polymerase); it enables the virus to synthesise DNA complementary to its own RNA, and this DNA is then incorporated into host chromosomes. Newly formed RNA results in new viral particles which, on release, may infect adjacent cells. A recently identified oncornavirus has been associated with human T cell lymphoma/leukaemia and designated HIV; in addition, HIV has been implicated in the acquired immune deficiency syndrome (AIDS). Certain RNA viruses also contain genetic information ('*oncogenes*') for transforming host cells. Oncogenes probably represent recombination of normal cellular genes ('*proto-oncogenes*'); when activated, they allow synthesis of new oncogene-coded proteins, some of which are related to growth factors and can, therefore, increase cell proliferation.

DNA tumour viruses become incorporated into cell chromosomes and replicate with host cell DNA. They cannot be detected in infected cells, but transformed cells can synthesise virus-coded proteins ('T antigens' in the nucleus and 'tumour-specific transplantation antigens' on cell surfaces). Although many DNA viruses cause tumours in animals, only one group, herpesviruses, is associated with human neoplasia. Epstein–Barr virus (EBV) has been implicated in Burkitt's lymphoma and nasopharyngeal carcinoma; more recently, herpes simplex virus type 2 (HSV-2) has been linked with carcinoma of the uterine cervix.

Genetic influences

Genetic influences are important in two ways.

An *inherited predisposition* to neoplasia can exist with retinoblastoma, neurofibromatosis, the multiple endocrine neoplasia syndrome (with neoplasms in thyroid and adrenal glands) and familial polyposis coli. Defective DNA repair mechanisms produce neoplasms in xeroderma pigmentosum, Bloom's syndrome and ataxia telangiectasia.

Chromosomal abnormalities may contribute to carcinogenesis by altering genetic sequences, and include point mutation, partial deletion, translocation (the Philadelphia chromosome 22 in chronic myeloid leukaemia is abnormal, part of it having become added to chromosome 9), re-arrangement and gene amplification. These processes may be important in oncogene activation.

OCCUPATION-RELATED NEOPLASMS

Since Pott described scrotal cancer in chimney sweeps two hundred years ago, many neoplasms have been caused by exposure to carcinogenic agents during work. In the cotton industry, skin carcinoma ('mule-spinners' cancer) was caused by mineral oil; bladder carcinoma in the rubber industry was due to aniline dyes; outdoor workers have a higher incidence of carcinoma of exposed skin; in asbestos works mesothelioma often follows apparently mild exposure, usually after many years; early radiation workers experienced carcinomas and leukaemia.

CLASSIFICATION

All tumours are classified in two ways—according to behaviour (i.e. whether benign or malignant) and histogenesis (the tissue of origin).

Behaviour

Important differences between benign and malignant tumours are summarized in Table 10.1.

Table 10.1 Differences between benign and malignant tumours

	Benign	Malignant
Growth	Slow; by expansion only	Rapid; by expansion and invasion
	Encapsulated	*Not* encapsulated
Spread	*Never* metastasise	Metastasise
Structure	High degree of differentiation	Variable differentiation from well differentiated to anaplastic.
	Regular cytology	Loss of polarity; cellular and nuclear pleomorphism
	Few mitoses (all normal)	Numerous mitoses (some abnormal)
	Necrosis—rare	Necrosis—frequent

Local *invasion* is an important feature confined to malignant tumours.

A *capsule* is a rim of fibrous tissue and compressed but otherwise normal adjacent tissue surrounding a benign tumour.

A *metastasis (secondary tumour)* is a tumour deposit remote from its site of origin (i.e. the *primary tumour*); benign tumours *never* metastasise. Spread of malignant tumours is considered separately later.

Differentiation reflects histological resemblance to the tissue of origin; benign tumours are always well differentiated, whereas malignant tumours can range from well differentiated to undifferentiated (where there are no features to indicate the cell of origin—that is *anaplastic*).

Polarity is the normal, regular, layered arrangement of cells.

Pleomorphism indicates variation in shape and size of cells and nuclei.

Necrosis occurs during rapid growth when cells are more than 180 μm from the nearest blood vessel (Chapter 11).

Histogenesis

Histogenesis indicates the tissue of origin; the majority are epithelial.

Epithelium. Benign tumours of surface epithelium are *papillomas* (e.g. squamous cell papilloma, transitional cell papilloma); benign glandular epithelial tumours are *adenomas.* All malignant counterparts are *carcinomas* (e.g. squamous cell carcinoma, transitional cell carcinoma and adenocarcinoma).

Connective tissues. Here too, benign tumours have the suffix *-oma* added to the appropriate tissue prefix, whilst for malignant tumours *-osarcoma* is added—see Table 10.2. Often, malignant connective tissue tumours are collectively referred to as *sarcomas.*

Lymphoid tissue. All *lymphoid tissue* tumours (lymphomas) are malignant (Chapter 21).

Naevus cells. Melanotic tumours are considered in Chapter 25.

Teratoma. A *teratoma* is a tumour, principally found in testes and ovaries, derived from totipotential cells; as such cells can differentiate along various lines, several tissues (e.g. skin, muscle, fat, cartilage, tooth structures and gastrointestinal epithelium) may be present. They may be benign or malignant.

APUD cells. APUD cells are part of the endocrine system. The term is derived from the initial letters of their most important properties—*A*mine *P*recursor *U*ptake and *D*ecarboxylation. They include chromaffin cells of the adrenal medulla, non-chromaffin cells of the carotid body, intestinal argentaffin cells, pancreatic islet cells and some anterior pituitary cells. APUD cell tumours (*apudomas*) include carcinoid tumours, thyroid medullary carcinomas, pancreatic islet beta cell tumours, and bronchial oat cell carcinomas.

PREMALIGNANCY

Non-neoplastic tissue abnormalities predisposing to malignancy are said to be premalignant. Thus, chronic gastritis predisposes to gastric carcinoma,

Table 10.2 Classification of tumours

Parent tissue	Benign	Malignant
EPITHELIUM		
Glandular	Adenoma	Adenocarcinoma
Covering/lining	Papilloma (squamous cell; transitional cell; basal cell)	Carcinoma (squamous cell; transitional cell; basal cell)
CONNECTIVE TISSUES		
Fibrous tissue	Fibroma	Fibrosarcoma
Adipose tissue	Lipoma	Liposarcoma
Cartilage	Chondroma	Chondrosarcoma
Bone	Osteoma	Osteosarcoma
Muscle—smooth	Leiomyoma	Leiomyosarcoma
Muscle—striated	Rhabdomyoma	Rhabdomyosarcoma
Blood vessels	Haemangioma	Haemangiosarcoma
Lymph vessels	Lymphangioma	Lymphangiosarcoma
LYMPHOID TISSUE		Hodgkin's lymphoma; Non-Hodgkin's lymphoma
BONE MARROW CELLS		Multiple myeloma; Leukaemia
NEURAL TISSUE		
Glia		Gliomas
Meninges	Meningioma	
Schwann cells	Neurilemmoma	
Nerve cells	Ganglioneuroma	Neuroblastoma
OTHERS		
Melanoblasts	Naevi	Melanoma
Placenta	Hydatidiform mole	Chorion carcinoma
Embryonic tissue	Dermoid cyst (benign teratoma)	Malignant teratoma

cirrhosis to hepatocellular carcinoma, ulcerative colitis to colonic adenocarcinoma and oral submucous fibrosis and leukoplakia to squamous cell carcinoma. There may be cellular atypia and disturbed tissue architecture (Chapter 9) which, if severe, is called *carcinoma in situ*, implying that it will subsequently proceed to frank malignancy with invasion of underlying connective tissue. Whilst many do ultimately invade, in some sites (e.g. oral cavity) the natural history is unclear, and some may regress to a histologically less sinister stage. Occasionally, malignancy may arise in a pre-existing benign neoplasm; examples include adenocarcinomas from adenomas of the colon and salivary gland pleomorphic adenomas, and sarcoma in neurofibromatosis.

SPREAD OF MALIGNANT NEOPLASMS

Malignant tumours are characterised by infiltration into adjacent tissues and the ability to metastasise. Several modes of spread are described.

Direct spread occurs at the periphery. Cells become detached, and move either actively by amoeboid movement or passively along planes of least resistance into adjacent tissues or structures. This includes spread along natural passages (e.g. bronchi and ureter) and along nerves.

Lymphatic spread, a common feature of carcinomas, occurs into regional lymph nodes. Tumour cells enter via afferent vessels, and are therefore found initially in subcapsular sinuses; eventually, the whole node may be replaced, and retrograde spread can occur.

Blood spread characterises sarcomas, but occurs frequently with carcinomas. Usually, tumour cells enter the circulation by direct local invasion of blood vessels, usually veins; less commonly, they may enter from lymphatics via the thoracic duct.

Transcoelomic spread occurs in pleural, peritoneal and pericardial cavities. A good example is gastric carcinoma spreading to ovaries, the most likely mechanism being gravitation to pelvic organs.

Widespread metastases to multiple organs is often called *carcinomatosis*.

GRADING AND STAGING OF MALIGNANT NEOPLASMS

Both are important in the routine assessment of patients with malignant disease as both are related directly to prognosis.

Grading is the pathologist's subjective impression of histological differentiation. Usually, the better the differentiation, the better the prognosis.

Staging reflects tumour spread at presentation. In general, the more extensive the tumour (e.g. into adjacent tissues, to regional lymph nodes and haematogenous spread), the worse is the prognosis.

IN VITRO CHARACTERISTICS OF MALIGNANCY

Malignant cells have several biochemical, structural and cell membrane differences from normal cells. These are mirrored in their in vitro behaviour, as they lose contact inhibition of proliferation, grow in reduced concentrations of serum, produce their own growth factors, show impaired differentiation and, exhibiting anchorage independence, grow as colonies in agar gels.

EFFECTS

Benign tumours

Benign tumours produce *local* effects, including anatomical abnormalities (e.g. swelling and ulceration). When hollow structures (e.g. stomach, bronchus, bladder and ureters) are involved, there may be obstruction, collapse and infection; local pressure by spinal cord and brain tumours may lead to sensory and/or motor disturbances; benign endocrine tumours can produce excess hormones and thus hyperfunction.

Malignant tumours

Malignant tumours, in addition, produce *general* effects, some of which may be designated paraneoplastic syndromes.

Weight loss is frequent; its extreme form is termed *cachexia*. Although exact mechanisms are not known, contributing factors include loss of appetite, malabsorption and the increased competitive uptake of nutrients by tumour cells.

Anaemia can follow haemorrhage from the tumour, impaired red cell production (from nutritional deficiencies or extensive bone marrow tumour deposits) or red cell haemolysis (haemolytic anaemia).

Thrombotic complications are particularly associated with certain tumours (e.g. pancreatic carcinoma). There may be multiple, transient venous thrombi involving different sites (*thrombophlebitis migrans*) or thrombi on heart valves (non-bacterial thrombotic endocarditis).

Neurological disorders, such as peripheral neuropathies and cerebellar degeneration, have been associated with bronchial carcinomas. Autoimmune mechanisms are probably involved, with the tumour producing antigens normally associated with neural tissue.

Muscular disorders (myopathies) also represent immunological reactions to tumour cell products.

Endocrine disorders are due to ectopic or inappropriate hormone production by tumour cells. *Cushing's syndrome* is associated with bronchogenic oat cell carcinoma which can produce adrenocorticotrophic-like hormones. *Hypercalcaemia* is common; it may result from widespread bone destruction by tumour deposits or from tumour parathyroid-like hormone and prostaglandin production (e.g. squamous cell carcinoma of lung). *Hypoglycaemia* may be associated with fibrosarcoma or liver cell carcinoma, both of which can produce insulin-like substances.

Finger clubbing (hypertrophic osteoarthropathy) is commonly seen with bronchial carcinoma.

Acanthosis nigricans, characterised by grey-black raised patches on skin and oral mucous membranes, may occur, especially with gastric carcinoma.

TUMOUR MARKERS

Tumour markers may indicate presence, progression and type of malignancy.

Serum markers include acid phosphatase (in prostatic carcinoma), Bence–Jones protein (multiple myeloma), carcinoembryonic antigen (CEA, in colorectal carcinoma) and adrenocorticotrophic, antidiuretic and melanocyte-stimulating hormones, parathormone and calcitonin (bronchogenic carcinoma). Frequently, as tumour volume falls, circulating marker levels decrease, thus providing a means of monitoring treatment effectiveness.

Cell markers can be used immunochemically to diagnose neoplasm type, and include common leucocyte antigen (for lymphomas), epithelial membrane antigen and oestrogen receptors (breast cancer), neurone-specific enolase (malignant melanoma) and immunoglobulins (multiple myeloma). Antibodies to cytoplasmic cytoskeleton intermediate filaments may indicate the cell of origin, as all epithelial cells contain cytokeratin, fibroblasts and mesenchymal cells contain vimentin and desmin is present in muscle cells.

11

Effects of radiation

Definitions
Ionising radiations
Mechanisms and sites of damage
Effects on cells
Radiation sensitivity assays
Effects on tissues

Non-ionising radiations
Ultraviolet radiation
Mechanisms and sites of damage
Effects on cells
Effects on tissues
Radiotherapy
Dental aspects

DEFINITIONS

Gray (Gy). The absorbed dose required to deposit 1 joule of energy/kilogram of tissue irradiated.

Rad. The absorbed dose required to deposit 100 ergs of energy/kilogram of tissue irradiated (thus 100 rad = 1 Gy; 1 rad = 1 cGy).

Linear energy transfer (LET). The average amount of energy deposited along each micron length of the radiation track (measured as kiloelectron volts/micron, keV/μm).

Relative biological efficiency (RBE). A measure of the biological effectiveness of one type of radiation relative to another.

D_o. The dose of radiation required to reduce the fraction of surviving cells (*f*) by one natural logarithm, that is to approximately 0.37*f*.

Types of radiation. Radiations can be divided into *ionising* (producing ions and free radicals within cells) and *non-ionising* (such as ultraviolet).

IONISING RADIATIONS

These include neutrons, α-particles (helium nuclei), β-particles (electrons) and short wavelength electromagnetic radiation. The last includes γ and X-rays, where ability to penetrate tissue is in inverse proportion to wavelength.

Mechanisms and sites of damage

The *target theory* postulates specific intracellular 'targets', damage to which causes cell death. The number of susceptible targets per cell may be one for viruses but several for mammalian cells. The higher the radiation dose, the greater is the likelihood that enough targets will be hit to kill the cell. In contrast, the *poison theory* states that ionising radiations produce intracellular free radicals which are biologically very damaging. High LET radiation (e.g. α-particles) deposits more energy along each track than lower LET radiation (e.g. γ-rays) and therefore kills more cells. At the tissue level, gross damage also reflects radiation type; thus the $LD_{50/5}$ dose (the dose required to kill 50% of animals by the fifth day after irradiation) for mice is 13 Gy for γ-rays and 6 Gy for neutrons (high LET radiation). Sites of damage include DNA, chromosomes (which may become fragmented and abnormal) and cell membranes.

Effects on cells

Effects on cells depend on both the cell's proliferative state and the radiation dose and type. Ionising radiation affects proliferating rather than non-proliferating, differentiated cells, a concept embodied in the *Law of Bergonie and Tribondeau*—'the sensitivity of a tissue to ionising radiation is inversely proportional to its degree of differentiation'. In practice, tissues containing rapidly proliferating cells are very radiosensitive—thus bone marrow and intestinal crypts are much more radiosensitive than brain. However, not all proliferating cells are equally radiosensitive—those in mitosis are much more sensitive than those in the DNA-synthetic phase (S phase) of the cycle. Irradiated cells may show the following changes:

Mitotic delay. Progression through the cell cycle is slowed, often by 1–2 hours/Gy.

Multinucleation. Doses less than 10 Gy cause breakdown in coordination of nuclear and cytoplasmic division to produce bi- or multinucleate giant cells.

Reproductive death. Many irradiated cells become capable of no or limited further division before ceasing, prematurely, to reproduce. Linked to this is *premature maturation* in which cells whose division potential has been reduced by radiation undergo accumulation of differentiation features.

Interphase death. Typically, doses over 100 Gy kill cells in even the most resistant part of the cell cycle. However, tissues such as intestine, skin and testis contain occasional proliferating cells that are killed by doses as low as 0.01 to 1 Gy; these cells undergo apoptosis (Chapter 2). Interphase death therefore occurs at very high and very low doses, even though mechanisms of damage are different.

Radiation sensitivity assays

The D_o value represents one measure of cell radiosensitivity. Typical radiation survival curves for X-rays and α-particles are shown in Figure 11.1. There is an exponential decrease in the surviving fraction with increasing dose (straight line), but in the X-ray curve this is preceded by a shoulder region, indicating a threshold dose below which cell killing does not occur; this is largely attributable to production of *sublethal damage* (SLD) which cells are capable of repairing. Absence of SLD is more common after high LET radiation, as even small doses deposit sufficient energy to kill the cell. The D_o value is the dose required to decrease the surviving cell fraction on the exponential portion of the curve by one natural logarithm (e.g. $D_2 - D_1$Gy, Fig. 11.1). For most mammalian cells, D_o values lie between 1 and 2 Gy; for epidermis and intestinal mucosa it is 1 to 1.3 Gy. The RBE of α-particles compared to X-rays is the ratio of doses required to produce the same biological effect (e.g. D_4/D_3 in Fig. 11.1). Such curves are determined by the most radioresistant tissue cells (i.e. those still capable of clonal division) and do not reflect the radiosensitivity of the most susceptible cells (i.e.

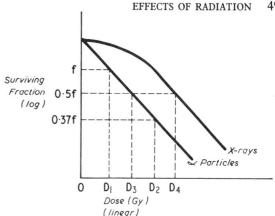

Fig. 11.1 An example of radiation survival curves for mammalian cells

those killed). Using apoptotic cells as the basis for in vivo assays, a D_o value of 0.1 Gy is obtained for mouse small intestine as opposed to 1 to 1.3 Gy obtained from classical survival curves as shown in Figure 11.1. Different subpopulations of proliferating cells in tissues such as epidermis, intestine, testis and bone marrow probably have a range of radiosensitivities lying between these two extreme values.

Effects on tissues

Whole body irradiation. A single dose above 8 Gy produces death, the timing of which is dose dependent. Over 50 Gy leads to brain damage (the *cerebral syndrome*) and death in 1 to 2 days; 8–50 Gy produces the *gastrointestinal syndrome*, with vomiting, dehydration, diarrhoea and shock, which causes death after 4 to 5 days. A single dose of approximately 8 Gy causes *bone marrow ablation* and death within a few weeks. Lower doses are compatible with recovery, but even 5 Gy will interfere with cell production in bone marrow, causing a decrease in circulating granulocytes, platelets, lymphocytes and red cells; anaemia, infection and haemorrhage follow, and a long time is required for recovery. In humans, the LD_{50} (i.e. the dose producing a 50% mortality) for untreated, acute radiation sickness is approximately 7 Gy.

Carcinogenic effects. Malignant tumours may arise in irradiated tissues, often after a considerable latent period. One of the earliest associations was squamous cell carcinoma in irradiated skin.

Further examples include leukaemias in many Japanese atomic bomb survivors, sarcomas in bone irradiated for non-neoplastic conditions and hepatic angiosarcoma in patients given Thorotrast® (an α-particle-emitting preparation of thorium dioxide formerly used in angiography and retained within the reticulo-endothelial system for many years).

Other effects. Many tissues show early and/or late radiation damage. *Skin* exhibits erythema, ulceration, pigmentation changes and epilation. *Connective tissue* changes include fibrosis, persistence of abnormal fibroblasts and arterial luminal narrowing by intimal proliferation (endarteritis obliterans). Normal *bone* mass increase by epiphyseal growth is prevented by doses over 10 Gy; heavily irradiated bone has a poor blood supply, and local infection (osteomyelitis) can spread rapidly, necessitating surgical removal, a complication known as osteoradionecrosis. Irradiation of *testes* or *ovaries* can produce partial or complete sterility, depending on dose; other germ cell effects include gene mutation, chromosomal rearrangement and loss of genetic material. Radiation damage will lead to *impaired wound healing*.

NON-IONISING RADIATIONS

Ultraviolet radiation

Ultraviolet Radiation (UVR) is the part of the electromagnetic spectrum between white light and X-rays. It is divided, according to wavelength, into UV-A (long wave UVR, 320–400 nm), UV-B (sunburn UVR, 290–320 nm), and UV-C (short wave UVR, 200–290 nm). Unlike ionising radiation, UVR penetration is directly proportional to wavelength, thus 99% of UV-C is absorbed by the epidermis, whereas the latter absorbs only 56% of UV-A, the remainder penetrating deeper into the underlying connective tissues. Biologically, UV-C is very damaging whereas UV-A is much less so. A parameter that accommodates the ability of UVR to cause variable damage is the minimal erythema dose (MED), that is, that required to produce skin reddening by vascular changes. For UV-C of 254 nm, one of the most damaging wavelengths, the MED in humans is 9 mJ/cm^2 compared with a MED of 13 J/cm^2 for UV-A;

thus, UV-A is over one thousand times less effective than UV-C. In humans, damaging effects of UVR are greatly diminished by filtration of UV-C in the atmosphere and of intermediate wavelengths by epidermal melanin.

Mechanisms and sites of damage

UVR absorption leads to direct excitation of electrons and chromosomal damage including breaks in DNA chains, DNA–protein interactions and abnormal DNA base linking (e.g. thymine dimer production). Much can be repaired by several DNA-repair enzyme systems; one, photoreactivation (which requires white light), involves thymine dimer removal.

Effects on cells

All proliferating cells are affected by UV-C. Apoptotic cells are frequently seen shortly after UV-C and -B exposure; mutagenesis and carcinogenesis may also occur. Although UV-A has little biological activity, except in extremely high doses, it is used therapeutically to treat psoriasis (a hyperproliferative skin disease—Chapter 25) in conjunction with oral psoralens, which form a loose complex with DNA; skin irradiation with UV-A of 365 nm produces a photoreaction between the psoralens and DNA, resulting in inhibition of DNA synthesis and cell death (PUVA therapy).

Effects on tissues

Effects on tissues are restricted to superficial structures, especially skin. Erythema, pigmentation and ulceration occur, depending on exposure. Chronic exposure may produce connective tissue degeneration, vascular dilatation and neoplasia, especially basal cell carcinoma of exposed skin (e.g. face and scalp); squamous cell carcinoma of the lip may also develop and, as might be expected, is more common amongst outdoor workers.

RADIOTHERAPY

The object here is to kill neoplastic cells whilst

sparing normal tissues as much as possible. For superficial tumours, small pellets of radioactive material can be implanted to provide an internal radiation source in the vicinity of the tumour, but for deeper neoplasms an external source of penetrating radiation is required. A major problem is that tumour cells more than 180 μm from stromal blood vessels are hypoxic (180 μm is the limit of oxygen diffusion into tissues) and much more resistant to radiation. Thus, a well-oxygenated 7.5 cm diameter tumour requires a single dose of 40 Gy, whilst if only 1% of cells is hypoxic, 80 Gy are required. A large malignant tumour is likely to have several necrotic foci adjacent to hypoxic but living cells and surrounded by a collar of oxygenated cells 180 μm wide. Hypoxic cells may account for as much as 20% of malignant neoplasms. It is possible to reduce radiation damage to normal tissues whilst obtaining maximal tumour destruction by the following:

Dose fractionation. Multiple exposures, each a few hundred cGy, are given over several days or weeks. Shielding of normal tissues by specially constructed moulds ensures that radiation is delivered only to the neoplasm and its overlying tissues. Advantages of fractionation include sparing of normal tissues, a progressive fall in the proportion of hypoxic cells as tumour size decreases, and recruitment of proliferating cells, temporarily out of cycle, into more radiosensitive states.

Increased oxygen tension. Increasing the pO_2 diminishes the proportion of hypoxic cells and also shifts survival curves for low LET radiation to the left; that is, the same cell killing is achieved with a reduced dose.

Increased body temperature. Tumour cells are more radiosensitive if their temperature is raised a few degrees.

Radiosensitisers. Drugs such as nitroimidazole render hypoxic cells much more sensitive to radiation, allowing a given dose to kill a greater proportion of cells.

High LET radiations with high RBE values. These are more effective in killing cells. Recent developments have involved production of other high LET radiation particles from sources such as the cyclotron.

DENTAL ASPECTS

Although there are no radiation survival curves or D_0 values for human oral epithelium, it would be surprising if they were not very similar to those for epidermis and intestinal crypt epithelium. Cell-killing potential of low dose radiation is also unknown for this site but is probably slight, as most dental radiographs involve 0.04 to 0.14 Gy. Effects of radiotherapeutic doses to the head for cancer treatment include complete failure of tooth development if tooth germs are irradiated, failure of root formation and eruption if radiation is given once individual tooth crowns have formed and xerostomia (dry mouth) following salivary gland irradiation, which may be complicated by rampant dental caries and recurrent oral mucosal infection with *Candida albicans*.

The most important complication, however, is osteoradionecrosis, particularly in the mandible. Patients who are to receive radiotherapy to the jaws should be fit dentally before the radiation regimen begins, otherwise grossly carious teeth may have to be extracted later from bone whose blood supply is impaired, thus increasing the risk of osteomyelitis; similarly, teeth with gross periodontal disease should be extracted and those with apical inflammatory disease should be extracted or root treated before irradiation.

12

Vascular diseases

Normal
Arteries
Congenital abnormalities
Atherosclerosis
Monckeberg's medial sclerosis
Inflammatory lesions
Systemic hypertension
Aneurysms

Veins
Varicose veins
Thrombosis
Capillaries
Lymphatics

Normal

Arteries are of three types:

Large or elastic, including aorta, common carotid and subclavian arteries;
Medium-sized or muscular, representing main distributing branches; and
Small, the terminal branches which supply arterioles and capillaries.

Arterial walls have three coats: *tunica intima*, a thin layer of endothelial cells separated from underlying smooth muscle cells by connective tissue; *tunica media*, interlacing smooth muscle cells (and elastic fibres in large arteries) separated from inner and outer coats by elastic tissue laminae; and *tunica adventitia*, a poorly defined zone containing elastic and nerve fibres as well as small nutrient vessels.

Veins also possess three coats, but each is less well defined.

Lymphatics are extremely thin-walled structures seen as endothelial-lined channels devoid of red blood cells.

ARTERIES

Congenital abnormalities

Congenital abnormalities usually occur as aberrations in course and distribution; recognition, therefore, is of particular importance during surgery. Abnormal communications between arteries and veins may arise as developmental defects, but can result from arterial aneurysm rupture into an adjacent vein (below) or from penetrating injuries.

Atherosclerosis

Atherosclerosis or *atheroma* is a disease of large and medium-sized arteries; the basic lesion is a raised plaque within the intima. These *atheromatous plaques* increase in number with age, and can cover entire intimal surfaces of affected vessels. Histologically, they may contain lipid-laden macrophages, proliferating smooth muscle cells, collagen, elastic tissue and extracellular lipid (mainly cholesterol) deposits; many, however, consist mainly of smooth muscle cells and fibrous tissue. *Fatty streaks* represent early intimal lipid deposition; they occur widely, and are even found in children. Although they may either disappear or remain harmless, they usually progress to atheromatous plaques, especially in coronary arteries.

Complications

Well-established plaques may undergo several changes:

Calcification, which may be patchy or widespread, producing rigid vessels;
Surface ulceration and *rupture*, to produce microemboli (cholesterol emboli);
Overlying thrombosis, which is very common;
Haemorrhage into the plaque, which may result in vascular occlusion (especially in coronary arteries— Chapter 13).

Effects

Effects are common, and include:

Ischaemia, from luminal narrowing by increasing plaque size;

Infarction, from vascular occlusion by superimposed thrombosis or haemorrhage into the plaque; *Embolism* of overlying thrombus or plaque fragments;
Aneurysm formation, following tunica media weakening and elastic tissue loss (see below).

Risk factors

Age. There is a close direct relationship between age and atherosclerosis.

Sex. Death from complications of atheroma (e.g. ischaemic heart disease) is much less common in premenopausal women.

Familial predisposition. This predisposition, represented by an increased frequency of 'heart-attacks' at an early age, occurs, but may be due to clustering of other risk factors (e.g. hyperlipidaemia, hypertension and diabetes mellitus), which do have a familial tendency.

Hyperlipidaemia and diet. High serum cholesterol levels are associated with increased ischaemic heart disease. In particular, elevated low density lipoprotein (LDL) levels appear to increase the risk, whereas high density lipoproteins (HDL) lower it.

Hypertension. This appears to accelerate atherosclerosis, possibly by direct physical damage to vessel walls.

Cigarette smoking. Smoking, particularly 20 cigarettes or more daily, is associated with an increased susceptibility to ischaemic heart disease.

Diabetes mellitus. Diabetics have a twofold increase in myocardial ischaemia.

Physical activity. Activity protects against fatal ischaemic heart disease; higher HDL levels have been found in such individuals.

Obesity. This correlates directly with ischaemic heart disease, probably largely because of its close association with hypertension and diabetes mellitus.

Stress and behaviour pattern. 'Type A' individuals, characterised by impatience, hostility and competitiveness, show a higher risk of ischaemic heart disease than the more phlegmatic, less competitive 'type B'.

Pathogenesis

The thrombogenic (encrustation) theory postulates that small platelet and fibrin thrombi aggregate at the site of endothelial injury and undergo organisation to form plaques.

The filtration (insudation) theory requires increased filtration, through endothelial cells, of lipids and plasma proteins; the lipids are taken up by smooth muscle cells, which proliferate to form plaques.

The 'reaction to injury' hypothesis incorporates parts of both the above theories. Endothelial injury (which may be related directly to hyperlipidaemia, cigarette smoking or hypertension) promotes local platelet adhesion and release of platelet-derived growth factor (PDGF). Both PDGF and macrophage-derived growth factor (MDGF) stimulate smooth muscle cells to proliferate and to synthesise connective tissue elements to produce plaques.

The monoclonal (mutagenic) hypothesis suggests that plaques begin with proliferation of a single, genetically transformed smooth muscle cell. Mutagenic agents include viruses, cigarette smoke products and cholesterol metabolites.

Monckeberg's medial sclerosis

Monckeberg's medial sclerosis involves medium-sized arteries and is characterised by ring-like dystrophic calcification of the tunica media. It is unrelated to atherosclerosis, rare below 50 years of age and often asymptomatic, as there is no significant luminal narrowing.

Inflammatory lesions

Arteritis, *vasculitis* and *angiitis* are terms used interchangeably, as more than one type of vessel may be involved. Arteritis may be produced by specific agents such as bacteria, radiation or trauma but the more important forms are of unknown aetiology and pathogenesis (although immunological mechanisms have been implicated).

Polyarteritis nodosa affects medium-sized and small arteries and arterioles. Early lesions are characterised by intimal and medial fibrinoid necrosis, with perivascular cuffs of inflammatory cells including neutrophils, mononuclear cells and eosinophils; established lesions are seen as mural fibrous thickening. Although any artery may be involved, damage to renal and coronary arteries is particularly important, as intraluminal thrombosis, with resultant infarction, may occur.

Although the aetiology is unknown, immune complexes have been demonstrated in some acute lesions, and possible antigens include drugs (e.g. sulphonamides and penicillin), microorganisms (e.g. β-haemolytic streptococci) and malignant tumours; almost 50% of cases develop in chronic hepatitis B virus carriers.

Hypersensitivity angiitis (sometimes also called *microscopic polyarteritis nodosa*) affects arterioles, venules and capillaries. Histologically, fibrinoid necrosis may be present, but the only change may be a cuff of inflammatory cells. Specific forms include Henoch–Schönlein purpura and the vasculitis associated with connective tissue disorders (Chapter 23) and malignancy.

Wegener's granulomatosis is a rare condition in which vascular lesions of polyarteritis type and extensive granulomatous chronic inflammation produce ulcerating lesions affecting mainly the nasopharynx; oral mucosa is occasionally involved.

Giant cell (temporal) arteritis is an uncommon condition, affecting elderly people, characterised by granulomatous inflammation of medium-sized arteries; temporal arteries are often involved. Clinically, there is usually throbbing pain along the affected artery with tenderness, swelling and redness of the overlying skin; there may also be headache, visual disturbances and jaw or tongue discomfort.

Systemic hypertension

Definition

Although no generally accepted criterion exists, a diastolic pressure above *90 mmHg* or a sustained systolic pressure above *140 mmHg* is usually required. Pulmonary hypertension is considered in Chapter 14.

Classification

Hypertension may be primary or secondary, and is either benign or malignant.

Primary (essential, or idiopathic) hypertension accounts for approximately 85% of cases. Although its cause is unknown, it is probably influenced by both genetic and environmental factors—hypertensive families exist, and hyper-tension is commoner in black populations; possible environmental factors include obesity, stress and dietary salt intake. It is commoner in females, and its incidence increases with age.

Secondary hypertension follows other diseases, mainly renal (Chapter 18) or occasionally endocrine (Chapter 19).

Benign hypertension is a relatively mild disease, and with adequate treatment is associated with a good prognosis.

Malignant (accelerated) hypertension produces a very high blood pressure—the diastolic pressure is often 130 mmHg or above. If untreated, death will occur in less than a year; even with treatment, morbidity and mortality are still high. Although it usually arises de novo, it sometimes develops in pre-existing benign hypertension.

Vascular changes in benign hypertension

Larger arteries initially show medial smooth muscle hypertrophy, but this is soon gradually replaced by fibrous tissue to produce dilated, thickened, rigid, tortuous vessels (*hypertensive arteriosclerosis*). Atheroma, promoted by hypertension, is usually severe. Intracerebral vessels may show micro-aneurysm formation, and in hypertension 'berry' aneurysms are more likely to rupture.

Smaller arteries and arterioles show variable luminal narrowing by intimal and subendothelial deposition of amorphous hyaline material (*benign arteriolosclerosis*). Although mechanisms whereby this material accumulates are unknown, it is probably derived from normal plasma constituents.

Vascular changes in malignant hypertension

When malignant hypertension develops in existing benign hypertension, appropriate vascular changes (above) will be found. When it arises de novo, larger vessels may well be normal, as it mainly affects small arteries and arterioles. These show intimal and medial cellular proliferation to produce a laminated, concentric, 'onion skin' appearance around a markedly narrow lumen; in addition, there may be focal mural necrosis with associated fibrin deposition (*fibrinoid necrosis*) and, occasionally, intraluminal thrombosis.

Effects

Benign hypertension may be asymptomatic, or may cause palpitations, dizziness or headaches. Ultimately, death may be unrelated, but there is an increased risk of cardiac failure, ischaemic heart disease and intracerebral haemorrhage; renal failure is uncommon.

Malignant hypertension usually causes headaches; visual disturbances due to retinal haemorrhages, oedema and exudates are frequent, and renal failure is the commonest cause of death.

Aetiology and pathogenesis

Hypertension reflects an increased peripheral vascular (arteriolar) resistance, but mechanisms responsible remain largely unknown.

The *renin–angiotensin system* plays an important mediating role. Renin, released into the plasma from renal juxtaglomerular apparatus cells, converts inactive circulating angiotensinogen into angiotensin I; the latter is then modified, by enzymatic action, into angiotensin II, a potent arteriolar vasoconstrictor. Renin also stimulates adrenocortical *aldosterone* secretion; this promotes sodium retention, which also contributes to hypertension by increasing circulating blood volume.

Aneurysms

An *aneurysm* is an abnormal localised dilatation of an artery or cardiac chamber. *Fusiform* aneurysms affect the whole vessel circumference, whereas *saccular* aneurysms involve only part of it.

Types

Atheromatous aneurysms are the commonest. They are often fusiform, and usually develop in the abdominal aorta below the renal arteries. Results may include thrombosis (with possible embolism to the legs) and rupture (causing retroperitoneal haemorrhage).

Syphilitic aneurysms are most commonly seen in the ascending aorta. Effects include local pressure (on bronchus, oesophagus, major veins or vertebral bodies) and rupture.

Dissecting aortic aneurysm is associated with medial weakness or degenerative change (*medionecrosis*), and develops when blood is forced into the media through an intimal tear. Possible complications include compression of coronary or renal arteries (with resultant myocardial infarction or renal failure) and rupture (producing fatal pericardial, mediastinal or retroperitoneal haemorrhage).

Berry aneurysms occur in medium-sized cerebral arteries, particularly in or around the circle of Willis, and are due to a congenital weakness of the vessel wall. Rupture produces subarachnoid haemorrhage.

Microaneurysms are associated with hypertension, and affect small arteries and arterioles, especially in the brain, where rupture causes intracerebral haemorrhage.

Mycotic (infective) aneurysms result from vascular weakening by inflammation, and often complicate subacute infective endocarditis.

VEINS

Varicose veins

Varicose veins are dilated and tortuous; they are produced by prolonged, increased intraluminal pressure, and are seen predominantly in superficial leg veins. In long-standing cases, ischaemia of the overlying skin can lead to local eczema and ulceration. In elderly patients, varicose lingual veins are common, and appear as irregularly dilated vessels on the undersurface of the tongue.

Thrombosis

Although two forms are described, distinctions are often difficult and irrelevant.

Phlebothrombosis is encountered mainly in leg veins, but can occur in the periprostatic venous plexus in males and pelvic veins in females. It frequently complicates surgical operations and prolonged bed rest; the most important sequel is pulmonary embolism (Chapter 8).

Thrombophlebitis indicates venous thrombosis secondary to inflammation. *Thrombophlebitis migrans* (multiple, transient episodes of venous thrombosis) may be associated with a carcinoma somewhere in the body.

CAPILLARIES

Hyperplasia. This occurs occasionally in granulation tissue undergoing unusual organisation—for example, in the *pyogenic granuloma* of skin and oral mucosa. Here numerous immature capillaries (as both sprouting buds and small patent vessels) are seen in a chronically inflamed fibrous stroma. Although the cause is unknown, they may become very large, particularly the type arising in pregnancy (the gingival *pregnancy epulis*); the latter often recurs if excised during pregancy, but after delivery, it becomes much smaller as capillaries close down and fibrosis develops.

LYMPHATICS

Lymphatics, with their widespread distribution, are important drainage vessels and therefore are often involved in acute inflammation (Chapter 3) and tumour spread (Chapter 10).

Acute lymphangitis. This occurs in vessels draining pyogenic infection sites, and appears as painful, red, subcutaneous streaks; there is usually an associated, painful regional lymphadenopathy.

Lymphatic obstruction. This can result in local lymph accumulation (lymphoedema). Causes include lymphatic or regional lymph node obstruction by malignant tumour cells, surgical lymph node removal, postirradiation fibrosis and, in tropical countries, parasitic obstruction (e.g. filariasis).

13

Cardiac diseases

Normal
Heart
Ischaemic heart disease
Rheumatic fever and rheumatic heart disease
Non-rheumatic valve diseases
Myocarditis
Infective endocarditis

Non-bacterial thrombotic endocarditis
Congenital heart disease
Cardiac (heart) failure
Pericardium
Pericardial effusion
Haemopericardium
Pericarditis

Normal

Size and gross configuration have both clinical and pathological significance. The average heart weight in females is 250–300 g, and in males 300–350 g. Normally, the right ventricle is 3–5 mm thick and the left ventricle 13–15 mm; any increase is due to hypertrophy, and causes cardiac enlargement. Normal heart valve cusps are delicate and translucent, and lack obvious vascularity; in mitral and tricuspid valves, thin delicate chordae tendineae originate from papillary muscles and are attached to the free valve cusp margins. Histologically, myocardial fibres contain uniform nuclei which bear a relatively constant relationship to cell size; variations in nuclear:cytoplasmic ratio indicate atrophy or hypertrophy. The endocardium consists of a layer of endothelial cells with a thin underlying connective tissue zone. Epicardium and parietal pericardium are composed of mesothelial cells lying upon fibrofatty tissues.

HEART

Ischaemic heart disease

Ischaemic heart disease (also coronary heart or coronary artery disease) is due to a reduction in myocardial blood flow following coronary artery narrowing by atherosclerosis; rarely, other conditions including arterial spasm are responsible.

Incidence

Incidence is high in certain countries (e.g. Finland, United Kingdom and USA), but low in others (e.g. Japan, Switzerland and Italy). These differences have been attributed to factors relating to atherosclerosis (Chapter 12). It is the commonest cause of death in males in this country.

Results of progressive coronary artery narrowing

Angina pectoris. This is characterised by chest pain extending into the left arm and neck, and is caused by transient cardiac ischaemia, usually during increased demand (e.g. exercise).

Chronic ischaemic heart disease. Extensive diffuse and localised myocardial scarring can eventually produce congestive heart failure.

Myocardial infarction

Myocardial infarction, the most dramatic effect of ischaemic heart disease, results from sudden reduction or arrest of coronary blood flow.

Incidence. This rises with age; most cases occur between 35 and 64 years of age, but it may develop in younger individuals with a strong predisposing factor for atherosclerosis (e.g. hypertension, diabetes mellitus and familial hypercholesterolaemia).

Causes. These include thrombotic coronary artery occlusion, haemorrhage into an atheromatous plaque and, rarely, coronary artery spasm.

Macroscopic appearances. It may involve the full thickness of the myocardium (*transmural*) or be limited to the inner portion (*subendocardial*), and is invariably seen in the left ventricle. Nothing is seen in infarcts less than 12 hours old; by 18–24 hours they are pale or yellowish, and surrounded by a rim of congestion; after 2–4 days organisation begins, and such areas are much more sharply defined.

Histology. Dead myocardial fibres undergo coagulative necrosis, and release locally such enzymes as glutamic oxalo-acetic transaminase (GOT) and lactic dehydrogenase (LDH); these enzymes then enter the circulation, where they can be measured and used to confirm myocardial infarction. Necrotic fibres show increased eosinophilia, cytoplasmic granularity, karyolysis and eventual nuclear loss; they are separated by oedema and an acute inflammatory cell infiltrate. A healed infarct is represented by fibrous scar tissue.

Complications. Arrhythmias, usually ventricular fibrillation, often result in cardiac arrest and sudden death.

Cardiac failure. Extensive infarction will produce acute or chronic left ventricular failure.

Mural thrombosis can occur on damaged endocardium, and predisposes to systemic embolism.

Rupture, with massive haemopericardium impeding heart action (cardiac tamponade), causes sudden death.

Cardiac aneurysm follows large infarcts which undergo gradual dilatation; they predispose to mural thrombosis and embolism.

Pericarditis develops after 2–3 days; it is often localised to the region of the infarct, but may be more widespread.

Rheumatic fever and rheumatic heart disease

Rheumatic fever is an acute systemic disease, occurring principally in children and young adults, which follows throat infection by group A β haemolytic streptococci. It represents cross-reactivity between host immune responses to streptococcal antigens and host tissue antigens, particularly cardiac; its importance lies in long term effects on aortic and mitral valves (*rheumatic heart disease*).

Incidence

Incidence and morbidity have declined considerably over the past 40 years. Most cases today are seen among those living under crowded conditions and without adequate medical cover.

Features

Acute rheumatic fever comprises pyrexia, painful and swollen joints, subcutaneous nodules and cardiac involvement (when all three layers may be affected—*pancarditis*).

Pericarditis is seen as a diffuse, fibrinous exudate—the so-called 'bread and butter' appearance.

Myocarditis, which if severe can cause acute cardiac failure and death, is characterised by Aschoff nodules in myocardial connective tissues. *Aschoff nodules (bodies)* consist of a central, eosinophilic deposit of plasma proteins and swollen collagen surrounded by giant cells (derived from cardiac histiocytes), plasma cells, macrophages and occasional polymorphs.

Endocarditis is the most serious aspect, since it affects the valves. In the early stages, valve cusps are swollen, red and thickened, and friable vegetations of platelets and fibrin can develop along the free borders. As organisation takes place, the cusps become fibrosed, thickened and contracted. Similar changes occur in chordae tendineae to produce fusion, thickening and shortening. These changes, together with commissural adhesions, produce rigidity of valve cusps which hinders blood flow (*stenosis*); when valve cusps fail to close completely, regurgitation of blood occurs (*incompetence*). In rheumatic valvular disease, mitral and aortic valves are most commonly involved. Ultimately, surgical treatment (including prosthetic valve replacement) may be required.

Non-rheumatic valve diseases

In *mitral valve prolapse (floppy mitral valve)*, there is ballooning of one or both mitral cusps into the left atrium during systole. Most individuals are asymptomatic, but may present with breathlessness, palpitations, chest pain or sudden death.

Calcific aortic stenosis occurs frequently with advancing age. The valve cusps become markedly thickened by fibrosis and extensive calcification. Outflow obstruction produces left ventricular hypertrophy; eventually, cardiac failure and sudden death can occur.

Myocarditis

Myocarditis can occur at any age, and may induce

heart failure and sudden death; usually, changes resolve completely, with no residual effects.

Types

Viral myocarditis, attributed to Coxsackie A and B, ECHO or influenza viruses, may follow days or weeks after the initial infection, which is usually in the lungs or upper respiratory tract. Histologically, there is isolated myocardial fibre necrosis and a predominantly lymphocytic infiltrate.

Toxic myocarditis is usually diphtheritic; appearances are as for viral myocarditis.

Non-infective myocarditis results from hypersensitivity reactions in systemic diseases of immunological origin—for example rheumatic fever and systemic lupus erythematosus (Chapter 23).

Infective endocarditis

Here, the endocardium, particularly the heart valves, is invaded by organisms, resulting in friable, infected vegetations. Often, there is a pre-existing cardiac abnormality (e.g. rheumatic valve disease, calcific aortic stenosis, congenital heart disease or a prosthetic valve), and causative organisms are present in the circulation. Infecting agents include *Staphylococcus aureus, Streptococcus viridans, Streptococcus faecalis, Haemophilus influenzae* and *Escherichia coli*; occasionally, opportunistic organisms (e.g. fungi) are involved. These organisms enter the blood during surgical operations, dental extractions, urinary tract instrumentation and intravenous injections (especially in drug addicts). Vegetations consist of fibrin, bacterial colonies and a few inflammatory cells.

Complications include congestive cardiac failure, vegetation fragmentation and systemic embolisation to produce septic infarcts which may eventually form abscesses, and valve cusp rupture causing sudden cardiac failure.

Usually, infective endocarditis is divided into acute and subacute types, but this is no longer a clear distinction; nevertheless, the subacute form is still well recognised, and because of its dental associations is documented here.

Subacute bacterial endocarditis (SABE)

This invariably affects already damaged valves.

The vegetations are usually large, friable and loosely adherent.

Clinically, patients often present with fever, weight loss and anaemia; occasionally, the first manifestation may relate to emboli to brain, heart or kidneys. Smaller emboli can cause petechial haemorrhages in skin and mucous membranes, and splinter haemorrhages in nail beds. Painful subcutaneous nodules in the palm, sole and finger tips can also occur.

Complications include congestive cardiac failure, systemic embolisation and mycotic aneurysms (Chapter 12).

Prevention is important in dental practice. Although a transient bacteraemia during dental extractions or deep scaling is common, it is difficult to assess the likelihood of developing SABE: the risk is slight but real, and requires prophylactic antibiotic treatment of patients known to have rheumatic or congenital heart disease prior to extraction or other surgical procedures in the mouth.

Non-bacterial thrombotic endocarditis

Non-bacterial thrombotic endocarditis is characterised by small fibrin deposits on valve cusps, but, unlike infective endocarditis, the vegetations are sterile, with no inflammatory reaction. It occurs in patients with debilitating diseases (e.g. disseminated cancer), and systemic embolisation with subsequent infarction may develop.

Congenital heart disease

Congenital heart disease is one or more structural abnormalities of the heart and/or major blood vessels. It affects 6 to 8 per 1000 live, full term births, and all are associated with an increased risk of developing infective endocarditis. Causes are largely unknown, although some follow maternal rubella infection in early pregnancy. Some forms are very severe and incompatible with extra-uterine life; of the others, the most frequent are documented below.

Atrial septal defect. This is probably the commonest, although it is invariably of no clinical significance. Rarely, however, it may allow a venous thrombus to pass from right atrium to left, producing a *paradoxical embolus*.

Ventricular septal defect. Small defects are well tolerated, but larger defects, which may be associated with other structural abnormalities, produce shunting of blood from left to right ventricles, eventually resulting in right ventricular hypertrophy and pulmonary hypertension.

Patent ductus arteriosus. The ductus arteriosus is the channel through which, during foetal life, blood passes from the pulmonary circulation into the aorta. Normally, it closes soon after birth, and is completely obliterated by 8–9 weeks. A patent ductus allows blood to flow from the aorta into the pulmonary artery, producing pulmonary hypertension, left ventricular hypertrophy and ultimately, if untreated, cardiac failure.

Coarctation of the aorta. This is narrowing of the aortic lumen between the left subclavian artery and the site of the ductus arteriosus. In severe cases, blood reaches the distal aorta via well-developed collaterals; there is left ventricular hypertrophy and hypertension confined to the arms, head and neck (i.e. proximal to the coarctation); blood pressure in the legs is diminished.

Fallot's tetralogy. This is the commonest abnormality causing cyanosis; it is characterised by four features: ventricular septal defect, overriding aorta (which thus receives blood from both ventricles), pulmonary stenosis and right ventricular hypertrophy. Without early surgical correction, death can occur from hypoxia and heart failure.

Cardiac (heart) failure

Cardiac failure occurs when the ventricular myocardium is unable to maintain an adequate circulation to meet the body's oxygen needs, and usually follows progressive deterioration of myocardial contractile function. Although the heart is a single organ, clinically significant left- or right-sided ventricular failure can develop separately; failure of both ventricles is often termed *congestive cardiac failure.* Failure is invariably associated with dilatation of the appropriate ventricle.

Left ventricular failure

This is usually caused by ischaemic heart disease, systemic hypertension or aortic valve disease;

occasionally, it develops when an increased cardiac output is required (e.g. thyrotoxicosis and Paget's disease of bone).

Effects. These are seen mainly in the lungs as pulmonary congestion and oedema; breathlessness is the main symptom, and is due to vital capacity reduction by fluid and blood within air spaces.

Right ventricular failure

This usually follows mitral stenosis and left ventricular failure, with increased pulmonary circulation pressure, but also occurs with some chronic lung diseases (*cor pulmonale,* Chapter 14).

Effects. These are seen systemically. In the liver, there is centrilobular congestion ('nutmeg' liver, Chapter 17); the spleen becomes congested and enlarged; hydrostatic pressure in the venous circulation increases, producing ankle oedema and distended veins (particularly apparent in jugular veins).

PERICARDIUM

Pericardial effusion

Pericardial effusion is fluid in the pericardial cavity; it is usually *serous* (as seen in congestive cardiac failure), but may be *chylous* (following lymphatic obstruction by malignant mediastinal tumours).

Haemopericardium

Haemopericardium (pericardial haemorrhage) follows rupture of a myocardial infarct or an intrapericardial dissecting aortic aneurysm. The blood accumulates rapidly, impairs atrial filling and rapidly causes death—*cardiac tamponade.*

Pericarditis

Pericarditis is pericardial inflammation.

Fibrinous pericarditis is the commonest; causes include myocardial infarction, uraemia, rheumatic fever and, rarely, viruses (especially Coxsackie B). The irregular, fibrin-covered pericardial surfaces present a 'bread and butter' appearance.

Purulent or *suppurative pericarditis* occurs with

bacterial or, occasionally, fungal infections. Organisation is usual, and this may result in extensive, dense, fibrous adhesions which may interfere with normal cardiac activity (*constrictive pericarditis*).

Tuberculous pericarditis is now uncommon, but may complicate mediastinal lymph node involvement. It also can lead to chronic constrictive pericarditis.

14

Respiratory diseases

Nose and accessory air sinuses
Inflammation
Nasal polyps
Tumours
Larynx
Acute laryngitis
Chronic laryngitis
Tumours

Lungs
Normal
Congestion and oedema
Pulmonary embolism
Collapse
Pulmonary hypertension
Infections

Bronchiectasis
Bronchial asthma
Chronic bronchitis
Emphysema
Diffuse alveolar damage
Pneumoconiosis
Tumours

Pleura
Pleural effusion
Empyema
Haemothorax
Pneumothorax
Tumours
Dental aspects

NOSE AND ACCESSORY AIR SINUSES

Inflammation

Inflammation of nasal mucosa (*rhinitis*) can be caused by viruses, bacteria and allergies; adenoviruses can also produce nasopharyngitis and pharyngo-tonsillitis—the 'common cold'.

Acute sinusitis usually complicates acute bacterial rhinitis, but may occasionally follow dental sepsis; streptococci are often responsible, and there may well be some associated sinus outflow obstruction. Rarely, the infection may spread into adjacent bone or the cranial cavity. As the roots of maxillary molar teeth are very close to the maxillary sinus, sinusitis here may simulate pulpitis.

Nasal polyps

Nasal polyps usually follow recurrent attacks of rhinitis. They are smooth and glistening, often multiple, and up to 5 cm in diameter. Histologically, they show focal oedema, mucous gland hyperplasia and variable infiltration by eosinophils, plasma cells and lymphocytes; numerous eosinophils suggest an allergic aetiology.

Tumours

Tumours can arise from either mesenchymal or epithelial elements.

Nasopharyngeal juvenile angiofibroma is a rare benign, highly vascular tumour which almost always occurs in young males.

Carcinomas are usually of squamous cell type, although in some the histological appearances can resemble a transitional cell carcinoma; they present as ulcerating and fungating growths. An undifferentiated tumour associated with a prominent lymphoid stroma, the *lymphoepithelioma*, is related to Epstein–Barr virus infection. The adenocarcinoma is very rare, but is associated with woodworkers.

LARYNX

Acute laryngitis

Acute laryngitis occurs with acute upper respiratory tract infections and, very rarely nowadays, in diphtheria; pharyngeal infection (e.g. streptococcal tonsillitis) may extend to the larynx.

Chronic laryngitis

Chronic laryngitis is common in heavy smokers; occasionally, it may be tuberculous (secondary to open pulmonary disease).

Tumours

Tumours are uncommon; patients usually present with progressive, prolonged hoarseness.

Benign tumours

'Polyps' are smooth, sessile nodules which occur most commonly on true vocal cords. They comprise loose collagenous but vascular stroma, and are covered by regular stratified squamous epithelium. They are related to heavy smoking and, as they are also commonly found in singers, have been termed 'singer's nodes'.

Papilloma, a true neoplasm, occurs as a soft friable nodule, usually on true vocal cords. Histologically, finger-like projections are covered by regular stratified squamous epithelium. Multiple lesions may be caused by human papilloma viruses.

Malignant tumours

These are mainly *squamous cell carcinomas*. They are usually found after the age of 50 years, more common in males, and associated with cigarette smoking. Most occur on vocal cords, but some are found on the epiglottis or in the pyriform fossa. They are usually small (less than 1 cm in diameter) and may ulcerate.

LUNGS

Normal

Lungs are constructed for gaseous exchange between inspired air and blood. Air enters via the respiratory tree—trachea, two main bronchi, large bronchi, small bronchi, bronchioles (which, unlike bronchi, lack cartilage and submucosal glands in their walls), terminal bronchioles, respiratory bronchioles, alveolar ducts and alveoli. Tissue containing clusters of three or four terminal bronchioles constitute a pulmonary *lobule*.

Respiratory passages are lined by tall columnar, ciliated epithelium and mucus-producing goblet cells. Ciliary movement aids removal of foreign material into large bronchi and trachea; mucus prevents drying of the mucosa by inspired air and traps dust particles. Neuroendocrine cells are also present. Alveoli are lined by *type I* and *type II pneumocytes*.

Pulmonary congestion and oedema

Pulmonary congestion and oedema, following an increase in pulmonary venous and capillary pressure, are seen in patients with left ventricular failure. In long-standing cases, numerous intra-alveolar haemosiderin-laden macrophages (*heart-*

failure cells) are present, and there may also be thickening and fibrosis of alveolar walls, producing firm, brown lungs (*brown induration*).

Pulmonary embolism

Pulmonary embolism is discussed in Chapter 8. Large emboli may occlude the main pulmonary artery, resulting in sudden death; smaller emboli can travel further into the pulmonary circulation and produce pulmonary haemorrhage or infarction.

Collapse

Collapse is an acquired condition involving previously expanded lung tissue.

Obstructive (absorption) collapse follows complete bronchial obstruction (e.g. by tumour, mucus, exudate or an inhaled tooth) and absorption of alveolar air.

Compressive collapse follows compression by fluid, exudate, blood or air in the pleural cavity.

Pulmonary hypertension

This results from increased pulmonary vascular resistance secondary to chronic obstructive or interstitial lung disease, recurrent pulmonary emboli or chronic left ventricular failure. Morphologically, there are atheromatous plaques in larger pulmonary arteries; smaller arteries show mural thickening and fibrosis. It causes right ventricular hypertrophy and, ultimately, failure.

Infections

Infections are very common. Respiratory tract infections, mostly viral, include the 'common cold', pharyngitis and tonsillitis (sore throat) and influenza. Lung infections (pneumonias) can be bacterial, viral or fungal.

Bronchopneumonia

Bronchopneumonia is characterised by patchy lung consolidation with a pre-existing acute bronchitis or bronchiolitis. It occurs most frequently in infancy (when there has been minimal exposure to various organisms) and in old age (due to lowered defence mechanisms); it is often a terminal event in patients suffering from debilitating diseases (e.g. heart failure or disseminated cancer) and is therefore a common postmortem finding.

Aetiological agents. These are numerous, and include staphylococci, streptococci, pneumococci, *Klebsiella* and *Haemophilus influenzae.*

Macroscopic findings. There are foci of acute suppurative inflammation which may involve one lobe but are usually multilobar and bilateral; in more severe cases, foci may become confluent.

Histology. Acute inflammation is seen, with pus in bronchi, bronchioles and adjacent alveolar spaces.

Complications. These include lung abscess formation, spread to pleural cavity (producing empyema) or pericardium and bacteraemia with distant abscesses. As the inflammation produces alveolar wall damage, complete resolution is unlikely (cf. lobar pneumonia, below), and healing is mainly by fibrosis.

Lobar pneumonia

Lobar pneumonia is bacterial infection of an entire lobe. In contrast to bronchopneumonia, it classically occurs in young, healthy adults, and affects males more commonly than females.

Aetiological agent. This is invariably *Streptococcus pneumoniae* (pneumococcus).

Appearances. It has a very characteristic natural history; four stages are described, although some overlap occurs.

Acute congestion (1–2 days) represents acute inflammation in response to the initial bacterial infection. There is intense capillary congestion and an alveolar exudate containing red blood cells, neutrophils and numerous bacteria.

Red hepatization (2–4 days) is characterised by a firm, red lobe resembling liver. Histologically, there is capillary congestion and dilatation, and alveolar spaces are filled with exudate containing fibrin, neutrophils and red blood cells.

Grey hepatization (4–8 days) is associated with progressive intra-alveolar breakdown of neutrophils and red blood cells, with continuing fibrin accumulation; the lobe is bulky, and often has an overlying pleural exudate (pleurisy).

Resolution (eighth day) follows progressive enzymic digestion of the alveolar exudate—it is either resorbed or removed by macrophages. The lung is thus dramatically and rapidly restored to normal.

Complications. These can occur, but are uncommon. Pleurisy may progress to empyema; an abscess may develop in the affected lobe; organisation may produce local fibrosis, but this is rare, as alveolar walls invariably remain undamaged; blood spread may cause meningitis, endocarditis or metastatic abscesses.

Pulmonary tuberculosis

Pulmonary tuberculosis is caused by *Mycobacterium tuberculosis* and characterised by focal granulomatous inflammation. It is discussed in detail in Chapter 5.

Primary tuberculosis occurs in non-immunized individuals. In the lung, the primary lesion (*Ghon focus*) is located subjacent to the pleura, usually in the lower part of the upper lobe or the upper part of the lower lobe; there is also marked regional (tracheo-bronchial) lymph node involvement, this combination being the *primary complex.* Once immunity develops, healing by fibrosis usually occurs; sometimes, particularly in childhood, there may be haematogenous dissemination resulting in *miliary tuberculosis* (with multiple small, tuberculous foci in many organs) or single organ involvement.

Postprimary (secondary) tuberculosis results from either re-activation of a primary lesion or re-infection many years after primary exposure, and usually begins in apical or posterior parts of upper lobes. Its course is variable—it may undergo healing, with scarring and calcification; it may spread gradually to other parts of the lung, giving *progressive pulmonary tuberculosis* with erosion of bronchioles and cavity formation; it may rapidly involve large areas of lung to produce *tuberculous bronchopneumonia* ('galloping consumption'); it may spread to regional lymph nodes; there may be haematogenous dissemination producing miliary tuberculosis. Although most cases respond to chemotherapy, long-standing secondary disease may cause amyloidosis (Chapter 7).

Fungal infections

Such infections (e.g. aspergillosis, histoplasmosis and cryptococcosis) are uncommon, and are invariably opportunistic—Chapter 5.

Bronchiectasis

Bronchiectasis is irreversible bronchial dilatation; it may be *cylindrical* (when the bronchi are affected along most of their length) or *saccular* (when the dilatation is localised and more pronounced). *Congenital bronchiectasis*, a rare form, follows defective bronchial development, and usually affects a whole lobe or entire lung.

Aetiology. The main factors are collapse and infection. *Collapse* usually follows bronchial obstruction (e.g. by tumours, enlarged lymph nodes, foreign bodies or mucus impaction; rarely, it may occur with asthma and chronic bronchitis). The retained secretions develop bacterial *infection*, with mucosal ulceration and chronic inflammation. There is gradual muscle, cartilage and elastic tissue destruction, with fibrous replacement; it is this loss of muscle and elastin which eventually produces the bronchial dilatation.

Complications. These include lung abscesses, haematogenous spread (producing metastatic abscesses, particularly cerebral), organisation (leading to pulmonary fibrosis and, if extensive, pulmonary hypertension and right ventricular failure), and, in long-standing cases, secondary amyloidosis.

Bronchial asthma

Bronchial asthma, an episodic allergic condition, is characterised by bronchospasm and production of thick mucus causing severe dyspnoea and wheezing; rarely, a severe, persistent attack (status asthmaticus) can prove fatal.

Extrinsic (allergic) asthma starts in childhood and is triggered by inhaled (e.g. house dust, pollens and cat hairs) or ingested (e.g. milk, chocolate, fish and drugs including aspirin and penicillin) allergens; patients also often have other allergies—for example hay fever, urticaria or infantile eczema. It is a classical Type I, IgE-mediated hypersensitivity reaction (Chapter 6). Histologi-

cally, bronchi may show mucosal oedema and congestion, goblet cell increase, mucus plugging, muscle hypertrophy and infiltration by eosinophils.

Intrinsic asthma occurs in older adults, and is usually triggered by respiratory tract infections. There is invariably no family history of asthma, skin tests for allergens are negative and there are no other allergic conditions. Both types of asthma may also be precipitated by non-specific irritants such as smoke, cold, exercise and emotional factors.

Chronic bronchitis

Chronic bronchitis is defined clinically as a cough with sputum production on most days for at least 3 months in the year and for at least 2 years; there must be no other possible causative chronic cardiopulmonary diseases.

Incidence. This is very high in the United Kingdom; it is an important cause of morbidity and mortality, and is more common in males and lower social classes.

Aetiological factors. These are mainly tobacco smoke, atmospheric pollution and occupational exposure to dust. These irritants stimulate mucus hypersecretion, which causes progressive airflow obstruction; recurrent bronchial infections arising in retained mucus also contribute.

Histology. There is marked hypertrophy and hyperplasia of submucosal mucous glands and a variable, often mild chronic inflammatory cell infiltrate; the epithelium may show squamous metaplasia, particularly in cigarette smokers.

Results. Unless causative factors are removed, there is gradual progression, with recurrent acute infections and emphysema developing.

Emphysema

Emphysema is the *permanent* enlargement of air spaces distal to the terminal bronchiole, and represents an abnormal destructive change.

Classification. This is based on the *lobule*, the area surrounded by a fibrous septum and supplied by three or four terminal bronchioles. Two main types are described.

Centrilobular (centriacinar or bronchiolar) emphysema affects predominantly the respiratory bronchioles; alveolar ducts and alveoli are largely uninvolved. This type is commonly associated with chronic bronchitis. *Focal dust emphysema* is a variant almost entirely confined to coal miners.

Panlobular (panacinar) emphysema is uniform enlargement of the whole lobule from respiratory bronchioles to alveoli. Markedly enlarged air spaces may project from pleural surfaces (*bullae*). Although this type usually arises de novo, it sometimes represents the last stage of the centrilobular form.

Causes. Tobacco smoke is particularly related to centrilobular emphysema (and chronic bronchitis)—some smoke constituents stimulate neutrophils and macrophages to release elastase, which damages alveolar walls; air pollution may have a similar effect. Serum α-1-globulin fraction is a potent inhibitor of proteases, and a genetic antiprotease deficiency (e.g. α-1-antitrypsin deficiency) will result in unopposed endogenous protease activity producing alveolar wall destruction and predominantly panlobular emphysema.

Effects. Emphysema, particularly the centrilobular type, causes poor blood oxygenation, cyanosis and dyspnoea. Chronic hypoxia leads to pulmonary hypertension, and, eventually, to right ventricular failure—cor pulmonale.

Diffuse alveolar damage

Diffuse alveolar damage is caused by a group of diseases which affect alveolar walls and where healing produces diffuse interstitial fibrosis.

Causes. These include drugs (e.g. busulphan), oxygen toxicity, dusts (e.g. asbestos) and rheumatoid arthritis; in about 50% the aetiology is unknown (*cryptogenic fibrosing alveolitis*).

Results. Initially, there is an alveolitis, with macrophages, lymphocytes, neutrophils and eosinophils within alveolar spaces. This progresses to fibrous alveolar wall thickening, which ultimately impairs lung function and produces pulmonary hypertension and right ventricular failure.

Pneumoconiosis

Pneumoconiosis describes occupational lung disease—the non-neoplastic reactions to inhaled mineral or organic dusts.

Anthracosis (coal workers' pneumoconiosis)

This follows prolonged coal dust inhalation.

In *simple coal workers' pneumoconiosis*, coal dust is evenly distributed around bronchioles, and there is no clinical disability.

Progressive massive fibrosis usually involves upper lobes, and is seen as irregular areas of black fibrous tissue with necrosis or cavitation. Tuberculosis is probably responsible for massive fibrosis developing in individuals with simple pneumoconiosis. Progression leads ultimately to respiratory failure or pulmonary hypertension with eventual right ventricular failure.

Silicosis

Silicosis follows prolonged inhalation of silica-containing dust, and is found particularly in quarry workers, stone masons and sand blasters. Its main feature is an intense nodular fibrous reaction to silica particles, mechanisms for which are unknown, but may include local silicic acid production, an immunological reaction or phospholipid/lysosomal enzyme release from silica-laden macrophages. Ultimately, progressive fibrosis leads to respiratory failure and pulmonary hypertension with right ventricular failure; in addition, many patients also develop tuberculosis.

Asbestosis

Asbestosis is caused by inhalation of asbestos fibres. The resultant pulmonary fibrosis is diffuse, and correlates with duration and severity of exposure. Mechanisms are unknown, but (like silicosis above) may include immunological reactions and local enzyme release. *Asbestos bodies*, which are 'dumb-bell' shaped and golden-brown in colour, are found histologically in the lesions and in sputum from affected or exposed patients. *Fibrous pleural plaques* are also related to asbestos exposure, and occur in the parietal pleura and the upper surface of the diaphragm. The main complications of asbestosis are carcinoma and mesothelioma (see below).

Tumours

Lung cancer (bronchogenic carcinoma) is one of

the commonest malignant tumours in Western countries, and is much commoner in men. During the last 40 years, its incidence has shown a real and dramatic increase which does not merely represent the consequence of an ageing population or more accurate diagnosis.

Aetiology

There is undoubtedly a strong positive relationship between smoking and lung cancer, and this is predominantly to the type and daily consumption of cigarettes; risks from pipe and cigar smoking are less. Atmospheric pollution from burning fossil fuels may be a contributory factor, and associated occupational hazards include asbestos exposure and radioactivity from cobalt and uranium mining.

Histological types

Squamous cell carcinoma (48%) arises from squamous metaplasia of bronchial epithelium, and adjacent areas may show epithelial dysplasia or carcinoma in situ. Most are located in main bronchi, and many are large.

Oat cell (undifferentiated small cell) carcinoma (18%) arises from bronchial APUD endocrine cells (Chapter 10). Most are hilar, highly malignant and metastasise widely; some are associated with ectopic hormone production (e.g. ACTH, producing Cushing's syndrome).

Undifferentiated large cell carcinoma (18%) is probably an undifferentiated squamous cell tumour.

Adenocarcinoma (16%) tends to occur more peripherally in the lungs, and may develop in scar tissue ('scar carcinoma'); it is not associated with smoking, and its sex incidence is approximately equal.

Effects

Effects can be local, with bronchial obstruction causing collapse, bronchiectasis and abscesses. Lymphatic spread is to hilar and mediastinal nodes; blood spread is common, with metastases found particularly in liver, adrenals, bones and brain. Unusual effects include myopathy or peripheral neuropathy.

Secondary tumours are common. Lungs are the main site for metastases from sarcomas, but involvement by disseminated carcinoma is also frequent.

PLEURA

Each pleural cavity contains a small amount of clear fluid for lubricating pleural surfaces.

Pleural effusion

Pleural effusion indicates an increase in intrapleural fluid.

Types

Types relate to causative mechanisms involved:

Transudates follow haemodynamic or osmotic disturbances (e.g. in cardiac failure and hypoproteinaemia), and the effusion has a low protein content.

Exudates follow increased capillary permeability (e.g. in pneumonia, tuberculosis, infarction, connective tissue diseases and neoplasia), and the effusion has a high protein content. As discussed in Chapter 3, exudates may be serous, fibrinous, haemorrhagic or purulent.

Empyema

Empyema (pyothorax) is intrapleural pus or purulent exudate. There is pyogenic acute pleural inflammation (*pleurisy*) which invariably follows direct spread from subjacent lung. It may resolve, but usually undergoes organisation to form dense fibrous adhesions which, if extensive, will obliterate the cavity.

Haemothorax

Haemothorax, blood in a pleural cavity, is usually the result of a ruptured aortic aneurysm (Chapter 12) or of severe direct chest trauma.

Pneumothorax

Pneumothorax is air in a pleural cavity.

Types

Spontaneous idiopathic (primary) pneumothorax occurs in young people (usually 20–40-year-old males), and the lung appears normal. The air is usually absorbed without complications, but there is a tendency for such attacks to recur.

Spontaneous secondary pneumothorax follows rupture of abnormal lung tissue and is associated with emphysema, asthma and tuberculosis.

Traumatic pneumothorax follows perforating chest wall injuries.

Results

Intrapleural air causes compressive lung collapse. This can produce significant respiratory embarrassment, particularly if other lung diseases are present, and it may be necessary for the air to be drained surgically.

Tumours

Secondary tumours are common, and usually represent direct or transcoelomic spread from lung or breast.

Primary tumours (mesotheliomas) are relatively rare, but are important because of their association with asbestos exposure; there is usually a latent period of 25–40 years, and the incidence is rising. The lung on the affected side is covered by thick, firm grey-white tumour tissue which may involve the entire pleural surface. It can infiltrate underlying lung tissue, spread to hilar lymph nodes and, eventually, metastasise to the liver and elsewhere.

DENTAL ASPECTS

The most important aspect of lung diseases is that many impair gaseous exchange between inspired alveolar air and blood; such diseases therefore render patients unsuitable for general anaesthesia in general dental practice.

15

Diseases of the mouth and salivary glands

Mouth
Introduction
Dental caries
Periodontal disease
Recurrent oral ulceration
Oral premalignancy
Oral neoplasia

Salivary glands
Inflammation
Obstruction of salivary ducts
Sjögren's syndrome
Neoplasms

DISEASES OF THE MOUTH

Introduction

The commonest oral diseases are dental caries and periodontal disease. They affect most of the population and are the main causes of tooth loss. Other important conditions considered here are recurrent oral ulceration, premalignancy and neoplasia.

Dental caries

Dental caries is loss of tooth tissue following acid and proteolytic attack by bacteria in dental plaque (colonisation of tooth surfaces and adjacent soft tissues by microorganisms in a carbohydrate and proteinaceous matrix). The earliest abnormality, affecting fissures and interdental contacts, is seen clinically as a chalky white spot representing demineralisation of enamel by acid. Decalcification proceeds inwards towards the amelo-dentinal junction and then spreads to undermine otherwise normal enamel; hence the area of dentine undergoing demineralisation increases. Acid in dentinal tubules stimulates odontoblasts and pulp cells to produce *dentinal sclerosis* (deposition of peritubular dentine) and *secondary dentine formation* (in an attempt to distance odontoblasts from the acid insult) and causes *pulpitis* (pulp inflammation). At this stage, no bacteria are present within enamel or dentine, and the enamel surface is intact. Eventually, the latter breaks down, bacterial invasion begins and proteolytic digestion of dentine matrix quickly leads to loss of tooth tissue. Pulpal changes associated with dental caries are considered in Chapter 3.

Periodontal disease

Dental plaque at gingival margins for a prolonged period produces *gingivitis*, the earliest stage of which is an acute inflammatory reaction. After a few days, chronic inflammation develops, which, at this stage, is a T cell reaction (Chapter 6). Clinically, the gingivae are red, oedematous and swollen; gradual loss of collagen leads to a disruption of gingival fibres. *Periodontitis* usually follows, with further collagen loss, apical migration of junctional epithelium and loss of bone around the tooth. Gingivitis and periodontitis can be stable, with slowly progressing tissue damage. However, conversion to a B cell lesion, with a decrease in lymphocytes and an increase in plasma cells, is associated with more rapid loss of periodontal tissues. Eventually, bony support is so poor that the tooth is lost. Although advanced periodontitis typically affects middle-aged and elderly patients, some gingivitis or periodontitis can be found in most young people.

Recurrent oral ulceration

Recurrent oral ulceration (ROU) is painful ulceration of the oral mucosa, lasting usually 1–2 weeks, which heals only to recur at intervals. It is common, affecting females more than males, and is divided, on clinical appearances, into three types.

Types

Minor aphthous ulceration. This accounts for approximately 80% of ROU. These ulcers usually affect non-keratinised areas of the mouth, especially lips and cheeks. They are small (under 1 cm diameter), and heal in 10–14 days without scarring. Typically, up to five ulcers are present.

Major aphthous ulceration (10% of ROU). Single ulcers, over 1 cm in diameter, affect any part of the mouth. Healing can be protracted and may lead to scarring.

Herpetiform ulceration (10% of ROU). This appears as crops of pin-head size ulcers. They may be very numerous and can affect any part of the mouth. Healing occurs quickly. Despite the name, it is not caused by herpes viruses.

Predisposing factors

Predisposing factors or diseases include:

Genetic and familial. A family history is present in up to 50% of cases. The highest incidence amongst siblings exists when both parents are affected. The HLA system might be implicated in these associations.

Immunogical. Immune responses probably play a central role. ROU is common in patients with B cell immunodeficiencies, and 40% of ROU patients have circulating immune complexes. Ulceration may be produced by deposition of immunoglobulins and complement components within the epithelium and/or a cell-mediated immune response to epithelial components.

Haematological. Fifteen to 20% of ROU patients are deficient in iron, vitamin B_{12} or folic acid, and there may be an associated anaemia. Improvement of ROU often follows appropriate replacement therapy.

Gastrointestinal. Only a small proportion of ROU patients have gastrointestinal symptoms, mainly small intestinal disease with malabsorption. Although only 2–4% of ROU patients have coeliac disease, up to 60% of patients with coeliac disease have ROU. ROU may be associated with Crohn's disease and ulcerative colitis.

Hormonal. As ROU may improve or cease during pregnancy, and as, in a small proportion of women, ulcers develop only during the luteal phase of the menstrual cycle, hormonal changes may sometimes be relevant.

Oral premalignancy

Several non-malignant oral mucosal lesions are associated with an increased risk of carcinoma.

Leukoplakia is a purely clinical term for a white patch which cannot be rubbed off or diagnosed as any other condition. A proportion of such lesions, after a period of time, become squamous cell carcinomas; overall about 5% do so in the Western world where this is more common in the floor of the mouth but very rare in the palate. Some are associated with tobacco usage, the form of which varies with country and social custom—cigarette or cheroot smoking, reverse smoking (with the lit end inside the mouth), tobacco chewing or oral snuff taking; in India, many relate to betel nut chewing. Histologically, in addition to a thickened stratum corneum which is responsible for the white clinical appearance, most show either no or little atypia. In some, however, atypia is marked, and if the entire epithelial thickness contains abnormal cells, the term carcinoma in situ (CIS) is traditionally used; occasionally, invasive squamous cell carcinoma is already present. There is no firm evidence to suggest that oral CIS is more likely to become malignant than leukoplakia showing less cellular abnormality. The natural history is unpredictable, but most are stable lesions which remain unchanged for considerable periods of time; some regress and even disappear, especially if the patient stops smoking.

Erythroplakia is a velvety red, often painful, area which may co-exist with leukoplakia. It is uncommon but sinister, as over 50% are squamous cell carcinomas and most of the remainder are CIS.

Submucous fibrosis is a common premalignant condition in India and possibly represents a reaction to dietary factors such as chilli. It produces dense fibrosis in the connective tissues of the lips and cheeks, and leads to difficulty in opening the mouth. The overlying epithelium is often atrophic, and in about one-third of cases squamous cell carcinoma develops. In India, 40% of patients with oral carcinoma have submucous fibrosis.

Chronic hyperplastic candidosis presents as a speckled, red and white patch often affecting buccal mucosa just inside the angle of the mouth. Histologically, *Candida albicans* is seen invading the superficial epithelium. If untreated, some progress to squamous cell carcinoma; if treated with anti-fungal drugs, most disappear, suggesting that they are caused directly by *Candida*.

Oral neoplasia

Oral neoplasia is often identical to that arising elsewhere. The commonest benign epithelial neoplasm, the squamous cell papilloma, is the same as that in skin (Chapter 25).

Carcinoma

Oral carcinoma accounts for approximately 2% of all malignant epithelial tumours in this country but up to 40% in parts of India. The commonest malignant skin tumour is the basal cell carcinoma (Chapter 25), but it is not seen in the mouth, probably because hair follicles are absent.

Squamous cell carcinoma (*SCC*), which accounts for over 90% of oral cancer, shows marked geographical variation in incidence. The highest figures, 30–33 cases/100 000 population, are in Newfoundland (mainly of the lip) and India; the lowest, 2/100 000, are in Japan. Figures for Scotland and Southern England are 6.9 and 2.5/100 000 respectively. Previously, the male to female ratio was very high, but it has reduced markedly during the last 50 years; this can be attributed partly to increased cigarette consumption by women, but the incidence in men has also fallen. In the Western world, 70% arise in the floor of the mouth and lateral borders of the tongue; the palate is the least common site. In outdoor workers, the lip is commonly affected. Only a small proportion arises from pre-existing (premalignant) lesions; the majority develop in clinically normal mucosae. Aetiological factors include smoking, alcohol (heavy drinkers have a 10 times greater risk), industrial exposure (e.g. cotton workers) and, in lip SCC, ultraviolet irradiation. Although most oral SCC are well differentiated, prognosis is poor when compared with malignant skin neoplasms. Between 1962 and 1967, the ratio of cancer deaths (D) to registrations (R) according to site was 0.04 for skin, 0.1

for lip and 0.6 for mouth. The further back in the mouth, the worse is the prognosis; thus for tongue the D:R figure is 0.8. Reasons for this poor prognosis include effective lymphatic drainage facilitating early regional lymph node metastases, late presentation and a tendency to local recurrence, particularly in the posterior part of the mouth. Another measure of prognosis is 5- or 10-year survival. For early lip SCC, 66% survive 10 years; this figure falls to 38% for well-established lesions. For intra-oral cancer as a whole, the figures are 35% and 10% respectively. Regional lymph node metastases at presentation adversely affect prognosis—without nodal involvement 67% of patients with tongue SCC survive 5 years, whereas with metastases 5-year survival is only 17%.

The *verrucous carcinoma* is an uncommon exophytic, slowly growing neoplasm affecting elderly patients, most of whom smoke or apply snuff in the mouth. It is characterised by slow infiltration of adjacent soft tissue and bone, and has no real tendency to metastasise; accordingly, prognosis is good.

Malignant melanoma is very uncommon in the mouth.

Odontogenic neoplasms

Odontogenic neoplasms arise from the epithelial and mesenchymal cells of tooth development. Usually, they are found in tooth-bearing parts of the jaws, but occasionally involve overlying gingiva. They are not restricted to young patients in whom active tooth formation is proceeding, but affect individuals over a wide age range, as jaws and gingivae may contain such residual odontogenic tissues as cell rests of Malassez and glands of Serres. Most are benign or locally invasive; few are frankly malignant with metastases.

The *ameloblastoma* is the commonest epithelial odontogenic neoplasm. It affects males and females equally, is commonest in the fourth decade and typically involves the posterior mandible. It infiltrates cancellous bone and eventually produces jaw expansion. Although it may invade locally and recur, it is unlikely to metastasise. Histologically, it is unencapsulated, with islands or strands of odontogenic epithelium resembling tooth germs.

Some mesenchymal odontogenic neoplasms involve cementum or dentine deposition (e.g. cementomas and dentinomas).

DISEASES OF SALIVARY GLANDS

Inflammation

Inflammation (*sialadenitis*) may represent localised effects of infection and obstruction, or may be part of a more widespread, systemic process (e.g. Sjögren's syndrome—see below).

Infections usually affect the parotid.

Bacterial sialadenitis

Acute sialadenitis is often due to diminished salivary flow allowing ascending infection along the main duct, usually by *Staphylococcus aureus* or streptococci; less commonly, it represents exacerbation of low grade, chronic infection. Predisposing factors include drugs, postirradiation changes and the now uncommon postoperative debilitation or dehydration. There is local pain and swelling, sometimes with a purulent discharge from the duct; fever and an increased white blood cell count are also likely. Complications include abscess formation and septicaemia.

Chronic sialadenitis is often also a complication of reduced salivary flow; in the submandibular it may follow calculus formation. Less frequent causes include tuberculosis and syphilis.

Viral sialadenitis

Mumps is a paramyxovirus infection which usually affects children. Typically, there is bilateral, painful parotid swelling lasting 1 to 2 weeks. Occasionally, submandibular glands are also affected; rarely, other organs, such as testis and pancreas, may be involved.

Cytomegalovirus infection is found in many infants at routine postmortem examination. In older patients, it is invariably subclinical, but may present symptoms in those whose immune system is suppressed by drugs, and other organs (e.g. kidneys and lungs) are often affected.

Obstruction of salivary ducts

In major glands, calculus formation is the commonest cause of ductal obstruction; in minor glands, trauma is usually responsible.

Salivary calculi. These are accretions, within the ductal system, of organic material including mucins, desquamated cells and bacteria, the whole mass having undergone calcification by calcium phosphate and carbonate deposition. They are seen in the submandibular duct much more often than in the parotid, and are rarely found in sublingual or minor glands. Blocked secretions may become infected and the gland painful, especially at meal times when secretion increases. Sometimes the calculus, if small, is shed spontaneously through the duct orifice into the mouth; sometimes it ulcerates into surrounding tissues; frequently it has to be removed surgically. Histologically, the gland may show patchy atrophy of acini, replacement by fibrosis and chronic inflammation.

Mucocoele formation. Minor salivary gland ducts in the lower lip may be damaged by trauma from incisor or canine teeth. At the site, a bluish cyst appears, enlarges and bursts, only to reform. These mucocoeles represent either leakage of mucus into adjacent connective tissues where chronic inflammation ensues (*mucous extravasation cysts*) or mucus retention within a blocked duct producing cysts lined by ductal epithelium (*mucous retention cysts*). Although mucocoeles are the commonest cause of lower lip swellings, minor salivary gland neoplasms are more common in the upper lip. Submandibular duct damage may produce a large cystic swelling in the floor of the mouth, a mucocoele variant known as a *ranula*.

Stomatitis nicotina. The palatal mucosa of pipe-smokers is frequently studded with small, red papules. These are chronically inflamed, minor salivary glands with dilated, partially blocked ducts; the red appearance is often enhanced by the white tobacco-induced keratosis that surrounds them. It is largely reversible once smoking ceases.

Sjögren's syndrome

Sjögren's syndrome comprises xerostomia (dry mouth), keratoconjunctivitis sicca (dry eyes and corneal keratinisation) and a systemic connective tissue disease, usually rheumatoid arthritis. Middle-aged women are most often affected, and have circulating antibodies to salivary gland duct cells as well as to other tissues such as thyroid and gastric parietal cells. Complications of xerostomia include difficulty in swallowing, oral candidal infection and rapidly progressing dental caries. Histologically, major and minor salivary glands show atrophy and infiltration by lymphocytes and plasma cells. Affected patients have an increased risk of developing a malignant lymphoma.

Neoplasms

Neoplasms are fairly common (approximately 3% of all tumours), and are almost entirely epithelial (Table 15.1). Approximately 80% arise in major glands, of which 90% are in the parotid and most of the remainder are in the submandibular; sublingual gland tumours are rare. Intra-orally, the palate is the commonest site. In the parotid, 1 in 6 tumours is malignant, but this 'risk' increases to 1 in 3 for submandibular and to almost 1 in 2 for palatal gland tumours; this is due to the variations in incidence of different tumours at different sites (Table 15.2). Histological classification is complex, although essentially the neoplasms are benign or malignant, and arise from glandular tissue (mainly ductal cells). Classification is important because of prognostic implications.

Benign neoplasms

Pleomorphic salivary adenoma (PSA) is painless, very slowly growing, and can achieve considerable

Table 15.1 Classification of salivary gland epithelial neoplasms

Adenoma
  Pleomorphic adenoma
  Monomorphic adenoma
  Adenolymphoma

Carcinoma
  Carcinoma in pleomorphic adenoma
  Adenoid cystic carcinoma
  Adenocarcinoma
  Epidermoid (squamous cell) carcinoma
  Undifferentiated carcinoma

Mucoepidermoid tumour

Acinic cell tumour

Table 15.2 Incidence of salivary gland neoplasms according to site (per cent)

	Parotid glands	Minor glands
Pleomorphic adenoma	85	50
Adenoid cystic carcinoma	5	20
Mucoepidermoid tumour	5	25
Others	5	5
	100	100

size. A capsule, often poorly formed, separates it from normal salivary tissue. The term 'pleomorphic' was used in Chapter 10 to indicate one of the characteristics of malignant cells; in this context, however, it has no connotation for malignancy. Instead, it reflects the pleomorphic (i.e. variable) histological appearances both within and between different tumours. The neoplastic cells are ductal epithelial and myoepithelial, and are arranged as strands, cords, sheets or even duct-like structures. In addition, the connective tissue stroma also exhibits a variable appearance, and usually contains collagen, elastic tissue deposits, chondroid (cartilage-like material) and mucinous or myxoid areas in different proportions. The capacity for connective tissue to show various components in an epithelial neoplasm probably reflects an interaction between neoplastic epithelium and non-neoplastic mesenchyme. Formerly, these tumours were called 'mixed salivary adenomas' as the connective tissue was also considered to be neoplastic; this view is no longer held, and the term 'mixed' should be used only as a synonym for 'pleomorphic' or 'variable appearance'. Care must be taken during their removal to ensure that enucleation is complete, as the capsule can be tenuous, and small tumour fragments may be left in situ and cause recurrence.

Monomorphic adenoma is uncommon, with a fairly uniform histological appearance which lacks the spectrum of changes characteristic of PSA.

Adenolymphoma (*Warthin's tumour*) is benign, and predominantly affects elderly males. It arises almost exclusively in the parotid. Histologically, there are cystic spaces lined by a double layer of cuboidal and columnar cells typical of duct epithelium. The connective tissue stroma contains a considerable lymphoid component and there is a well-formed capsule.

Carcinomas

Carcinomas are rapidly growing, painful, and often fixed to surrounding tissues. There may be local bleeding, ulceration of overlying skin or oral mucosa and, in palatal lesions, resorption of underlying bone. Perineural lymphatic invasion often indicates an advanced lesion with metastatic spread. In the parotid, 25% of adenoid cystic carcinomas (see below) infiltrate and spread along branches of the facial (VII) nerve to produce facial paralysis.

Carcinoma in pleomorphic adenoma. Long-standing pleomorphic adenomas (usually over 10 years duration) sometimes undergo painful, rapid growth, with fixation to surrounding structures indicating malignant transformation. Affected patients usually die from metastatic disease within 1 year.

Adenoid cystic carcinoma. This is very common in minor salivary glands and has a rather poor prognosis, with only 13% of patients surviving for 20 years. Histologically, it shows characteristic islands of small, darkly staining basaloid cells containing cystic spaces—the 'Swiss cheese' or 'cribriform' appearance.

Other carcinomas. These are uncommon. They include the *adenocarcinoma*, which forms duct-like structures, the *epidermoid (squamous cell) carcinoma* and the *undifferentiated carcinoma*.

Mucoepidermoid and acinic cell tumours

Most neoplasms can be classified as benign or malignant by histological appearances. The behaviour of these two, however, is impossible to predict from histology alone; some are benign, whilst others are aggressive with recurrence and metastases.

16

Alimentary diseases

Oesophagus
Normal
Inflammation
Varices
Obstruction
Hiatus hernia
Tumours

Stomach
Normal
Inflammation
Peptic ulceration
Tumours

Intestines
Normal
Inflammation
Malabsorption
Diverticular disease
Intestinal obstruction
Tumours

Peritoneum
Normal
Inflammation
Ascites
Tumours
Dental aspects

OESOPHAGUS

Normal

The oesophagus is a muscular tube, approximately 25 cm (10 in) long, joining the pharynx and stomach and lined by non-keratinising squamous epithelium.

Inflammation

Oesophagitis due to infection is very uncommon, but opportunistic infections by low virulence organisms (e.g. *Candida albicans*) may occur in patients with depressed natural immunity. The commonest cause of oesophagitis is reflux of gastric juices; it usually affects the lower third, and may be associated with overt ulceration (see peptic ulceration below).

Varices

The submucosal veins around the cardio-oesophageal junction are one of the anastomotic sites between portal and systemic venous circulations. When portal venous pressure rises significantly (as in portal hypertension in liver disease—Chapter 17), these veins dilate and usually rupture into the lumen; this bleeding may be mild, but is often severe and frequently fatal.

Obstruction

As with any hollow tubular organ, oesophageal obstruction may be intraluminal, intramural or extramural, and will produce difficulty in swallowing (*dysphagia*).

Intraluminal

This is uncommon, but may be due to a swallowed foreign body.

Intramural

Tumours cause dysphagia, either by luminal obstruction or by infiltrating and thickening the wall. Stricture by excess fibrosis may follow peptic ulceration, accidental or intentional (e.g. suicidal attempt) ingestion of corrosive acids or alkalis or direct trauma; it may also occur with progressive systemic sclerosis.

Extramural

Extramural obstruction is also uncommon; it may be produced by mediastinal or bronchial tumours, aortic arch malformations, aortic aneurysms and thyroid goitres.

Neuromuscular dysfunction

Neuromuscular dysfunction will produce dysphagia.
  Paterson–Kelly (Plummer–Vinson) syndrome affects the upper end; it occurs in women with iron deficiency anaemia. No structural abnormality is found, but an upper oesophageal 'web' may be seen radiologically.
  Achalasia of the cardia (cardiospasm) affects the lower end. The cardia is markedly thickened and

narrowed, and the proximal oesophagus is dilated and hypertrophic.

Hiatus hernia

Hiatus hernia is herniation of part of the gastric fundus into the posterior mediastinum through the oesophageal hiatus. The aetiology is unknown. The condition, which is fairly common, is often asymptomatic, but there may be associated incompetence of cardio-oesophageal sphincter mechanisms with reflux of acidic gastric juice producing chronic peptic oesophagitis, ulceration, fibrosis with stricture formation or haemorrhage.

Tumours

Oesophageal carcinoma is fairly common and accounts for approximately 0.2% of all malignant disease throughout the body. It usually arises in the middle third and often develops between 50 and 70 years of age. Overall, it is much commoner in men, but in the postcricoid region, where a definite association with the Paterson–Kelly syndrome exists, it is slightly more common in women. As the oesophagus is lined by squamous epithelium, the tumour is invariably a *squamous cell carcinoma*, and often it is poorly differentiated. Direct spread to adjacent mediastinal components and lymphatic and haematogenous metastases occur early, and prognosis therefore is very poor. Other oesophageal tumours, both benign and malignant, are very rare.

STOMACH

Normal

The stomach is a muscular sac capable of considerable physiological dilatation. Its mucosa contains specialised glands secreting acid and enzymes to initiate digestion.

Inflammation

Inflammation here, as elsewhere, may be acute or chronic.

Acute gastritis. Most bacteria are rapidly destroyed by acidic gastric secretions, and

bacterial infection is therefore extremely rare. However, bacterial toxins (e.g. staphylococcal enterotoxin) and viruses (e.g. rotavirus) are often responsible for transient acute gastritis or gastroenteritis, and irritants (e.g. alcohol and aspirin) may produce similar changes. These comprise mucosal and submucosal congestion, oedema and polymorph infiltration; superficial mucosal ulceration is common. Regeneration is invariably rapid and total.

Chronic gastritis. This is fairly common. It may be focal and related, in a rather non-specific way, to chronic excess alcohol ingestion, heavy smoking or bile reflux, or it may be diffuse and autoimmune in nature.

Autoimmune gastritis. This is a progressive process. Initially, only superficial chronic inflammation is seen, but gradually the specialised epithelial glandular cells are destroyed and replaced by simpler mucus-secreting epithelium. Ultimately, the mucosa is considerably reduced in thickness and consists almost entirely of mucous glands (*atrophic gastritis* or *gastric atrophy*). As glandular destruction progresses, acid secretion is reduced (*hypochlorhydria*) and finally disappears (*achlorhydria*); similarly, in the later stages, intrinsic factor secretion declines, and megaloblastic anaemia due to vitamin B_{12} deficiency (Chapter 20) develops. Autoimmune gastritis usually occurs in middle-aged and elderly women; it may be associated with other autoimmune diseases such as thyroiditis, and may progress to neoplasia (see below).

Peptic ulceration

Peptic ulceration may be acute, but is usually chronic. It may occur wherever gastrointestinal tract epithelium is exposed to acidic gastric juices, and is therefore found not only in the stomach but also in the first part of the duodenum, the oesophagus, Meckel's diverticula and jejunum adjacent to gastro-enterostomy sites.

Acute

Acute peptic ulceration is often multiple and superficial, and may be associated with causes of acute gastritis (above), extensive burns and corticosteroid therapy. Rapid and total healing invariably occurs.

Chronic

Chronic peptic ulceration is very common, particularly in middle age groups and in men (M:F about 3:1).

Aetiology and pathogenesis. These are complex and largely unknown, and both genetic (as blood group O) and environmental (as cigarette smoking) factors contribute. Gastric acid is obviously very important—ulceration does not occur with achlorhydria, whereas acid hypersecretion is often associated with duodenal ulceration.

Site. Nowadays, duodenal ulcers are about six times commoner than gastric ulcers; chronic peptic ulceration elsewhere is relatively uncommon, constituting less than 3%. Chronic gastric ulcers are usually found either on the lesser curvature or in the pylorus; chronic duodenal ulcers are invariably within the proximal centimetre of the duodenum.

Macroscopic findings. Any chronic peptic ulcer may be quite large, but the majority are less than 3 cm in maximum diameter, round or oval in shape with steep sides and a punched-out appearance.

Microscopic findings. The ulcer base consists of granulation tissue overlying fibrous tissue, which usually replaces the muscle coat; marginal epithelial proliferation representing attempted regeneration is also seen.

Results and complications. Healing by fibrosis with restoration of overlying epithelial continuity usually occurs, although excess fibrous scar tissue may produce deformity and, especially with pyloric ulcers, obstruction. Recurrence after healing is common (almost 50%). There are three important complications:

Haemorrhage is due to erosion of one or more blood vessels at the ulcer base. It is very common, and usually mild; occasionally, it is severe; rarely it is massive and fatal.

Perforation is due to full thickness bowel wall destruction, and produces acute peritonitis.

Malignancy develops, in about 1% of cases, at the edge of chronic gastric ulcers; malignant change does not occur in peptic ulcers elsewhere.

Tumours

Benign tumours, both epithelial (adenoma) and connective tissue (e.g. leiomyoma), are rare. The commonest tumour by far is the *gastric adenocarcinoma*, which accounts for approximately 15% of all malignant disease. It usually develops between 50 and 70 years of age and is more common in men (M:F about 2:1). No definite aetiological factors are recognised, but both genetic (as blood group A) and environmental (e.g. diet and cooking methods) factors may apply. Two premalignant lesions are known—autoimmune gastritis and chronic peptic ulceration (above). Approximately half arise in or around the pylorus; they may project into the lumen or infiltrate extensively into the wall with or without overlying ulceration. Tumour spread (local into gastric muscle, serosa and peritoneum; lymphatic and haematogenous) is early and extensive, and prognosis, therefore, is poor—only about 10% are alive at 5 years.

INTESTINES

Normal

The intestines are approximately 7.5 metres (25 ft) in length, and extend from stomach to anus. They comprise small intestine (duodenum, jejunum and ileum) and large intestine (caecum with appendix, ascending, transverse, descending and sigmoid colon and rectum). In the small intestine, digestion of food continues and almost all absorption occurs; in the large intestine, faeces are formed and water absorption is completed.

Inflammation

As numerous bacteria normally colonise the intestines, infection and subsequent inflammation often complicate most intestinal lesions. In addition, several pathogenic organisms, when ingested, will initiate specific acute and/or chronic inflammatory diseases—for example *Salmonella typhi* (typhoid fever), *Vibrio cholerae* (cholera), *Shigella* species (bacillary dysentery), *Entamoeba histolytica* (amoebic dysentery) and *Mycobacterium tuberculosis*.

Acute appendicitis, acute inflammation of the vermiform appendix, is extremely common, particularly in children and young adults. Its exact aetiology is uncertain, but luminal obstruction is probably relevant. It is important because, if not treated by surgical removal, local spread to produce an appendix abscess or generalised acute peritonitis will probably occur.

Crohn's disease is relatively uncommon, although its frequency is increasing. Its aetiology remains unknown. Any part of the gastrointestinal tract, from mouth to anus, may be affected; in younger adults it is usually the terminal ileum which is most severely involved, whereas in elderly patients the disease may be confined to the colon. Characteristically, bowel lesions are multiple, with apparently normal, unaffected segments separating abnormal areas ('skip lesions'). Macroscopically, the diseased bowel shows marked mural thickening with associated luminal narrowing and a fissuring type of mucosal ulceration, which often presents a characteristic 'cobblestone' appearance. Histologically, there is marked submucosal oedema and fibrosis, with a chronic inflammatory cell infiltrate throughout all the layers of the bowel wall; in approximately 60% of cases non-caseating granulomata are also seen. The course of Crohn's disease is both variable and unpredictable—it may remit completely and permanently, but often it is protracted, with multiple remissions and relapses; occasionally, it is progressive and ultimately fatal. Complications include intestinal obstruction, fistulae (to other parts of the bowel or to external surfaces) and malabsorption.

Ulcerative colitis is more common than Crohn's disease; it is also increasing in frequency and its aetiology remains unknown. It usually presents initially between 20 and 40 years of age. It is confined to the colon; it may be limited to the sigmoid and rectum, but in almost half the cases the whole colon is involved. There is irregular mucosal congestion, haemorrhage and ulceration; histological examination also shows acute and chronic inflammatory cell infiltration, but, unlike Crohn's disease, the changes are confined to the mucosa and granulomata are never seen. The prognosis is also variable and unpredictable—a few mild cases may remit permanently; many run a prolonged, fluctuating course with numerous remissions and relapses; some have continuous disease; a few develop a rapidly progressive, fulminating disease which, without surgical total colectomy, is soon fatal, usually from severe haemorrhage, electrolyte disturbances and perforation. The major long term complication is malignancy, particularly with total colonic involvement and continuous disease for over 10 years.

Malabsorption

When the overall absorptive surface area of the small intestine is significantly reduced by disease, absorption of various digestion products and nutrients will be impaired and deficiency states will develop. As different nutrients are absorbed most effectively at different sites, the type and combination of deficiencies will depend on extent, location and severity of disease, but may include vitamins, minerals, proteins, salts and fats. Major causes of malabsorption include coeliac disease (see below), Crohn's disease (particularly with internal fistulae or following extensive surgical resection—see above) and chronic pancreatic or biliary diseases (Chapter 17).

Coeliac disease is related to *gluten*, a protein in wheat, and probably represents a genetically linked abnormal immune response. There is variable flattening, broadening and fusion of small intestinal villi (*villous atrophy*) due to reduced epithelial cell survival; compensatory crypt hyperplasia is present, and the mucosa contains an excess of chronic inflammatory cells. These changes are reversed by withdrawing gluten from the diet.

Diverticular disease

A diverticulum is a mucosa-lined sac in continuity with the bowel lumen.

Meckel's diverticulum is a congenital abnormality due to persistence of the omphalomesenteric duct. It is found in approximately 2% of the population about 60 cm (2 ft) proximal to the ileocaecal valve. It is usually asymptomatic, but, because the mucosa may contain heterotopic gastric and/or pancreatic epithelium, peptic ulceration, bleeding or even perforation may occur. Other small intestinal diverticula are rare.

Diverticulosis is multiple diverticula in the large intestine. It is very common, being present, to some extent, in about 20% of elderly patients; invariably the sigmoid colon is affected most severely. Diverticulosis is related to high intra-luminal pressures and to a relative deficiency of dietary roughage. The diverticular mucosa herniates through weak points in the colonic muscular wall between the three longitudinal bands of muscle fibres (taeniae coli) and at the entry sites of blood vessels. Usually, diverticulosis is asymptomatic, but in about 20% of cases diverticulitis supervenes.

Diverticulitis is inflammation of pre-existing diverticulosis. Initially, the inflammation is acute, and may spread to produce local abscess forma-tion, generalised acute peritonitis or fistulae with adjacent organs. Later, the inflammation may become chronic, with mural fibrosis causing luminal obstruction. Another important compli-cation is acute or chronic haemorrhage.

Intestinal obstruction

Intestinal obstruction (ileus), impaired passage of intestinal contents, may be partial or complete and due to intraluminal, intramural, extramural or paralytic factors.

Intraluminal

Intraluminal causes include swallowed foreign bodies, gallstones and inspissated meconium in fibrocystic disease (Chapter 17).

Intramural

Intramural lesions include tumours, Crohn's disease, diverticulitis and various congenital abnormalities.

Intussusception is invagination of a bowel segment into the immediately distal intestinal lumen. It invariably involves the small intestine and usually occurs in children; occasionally, a benign tumour or enlarged intestinal lymphoid tissue is present at the apex of the intussusception. The invaginated bowel wall blood supply is compressed, with subsequent ischaemia and infarction as well as obstruction.

Extramural

Fibrous adhesions following localised inflam-mation or surgery and adjacent tumours may compress the bowel to produce obstruction.

Hernias, where bowel protrudes outside the normal peritoneal cavity confines (e.g. in inguinal or femoral canals), cause obstruction if strangu-lation occurs—that is, when the bowel becomes impacted and its blood supply impaired.

Volvulus involves bowel rotation through at least 180°; this produces obstruction and vascular compression with ischaemia and infarction. It may occur in the small intestine, but more commonly affects the sigmoid colon.

Paralytic ileus

Paralytic ileus indicates impaired bowel motility without mechanical obstruction. It occurs tran-siently after most abdominal surgery and may follow acute generalised peritonitis, severe ab-dominal trauma, severe toxaemia or superior mesenteric vascular occlusion by thrombosis or embolism.

Tumours

Tumours of the small intestine are rare, and account for only about 0.2% of all deaths from malignant disease; most are carcinoid tumours (Chapter 10). In contrast, large intestine tumours are very common.

Adenomatous polyps

Adenomatous polyps are benign epithelial neoplasms, and almost 5% of adults develop such tumours. They occur most commonly in the sigmoid colon and rectum, and are frequently multiple. Their importance lies in the high risk of subsequent malignant change.

Familial polyposis coli is an hereditary condition associated with innumerable adenomatous polyps.

Gardner's syndrome comprises multiple adenom-atous polyps together with skin abnormalities, osteomas of the jaw and skull and unerupted supernumary teeth.

Peutz–Jeghers syndrome

The Peutz–Jeghers syndrome is a rare autosomal dominant hereditary disorder consisting of multiple polyps, most of which are in the small intestine, and pigmented lesions on lips, mouth and digits. The polyps are probably hamartomatous (i.e. developmental abnormalities) rather than neoplastic; they are usually asymptomatic, but may cause intussusception or chronic blood loss.

Adenocarcinoma

Adenocarcinoma of the large bowel is one of the commonest of all malignancies and accounts for almost 16% of deaths from malignant disease. It usually develops between 55 and 65 years of age, and has an equal sex incidence. Just over one-third arise in the rectum and rectosigmoid region; sigmoid colon and caecum are the other common sites. The aetiology remains unknown, although adenomatous polyps (including those associated with familial polyposis coli and Gardner's syndrome) and long-standing continuous ulcerative colitis are recognised predisposing conditions. These tumours tend to be polypoid, and often involve the entire circumference of the bowel wall to produce luminal narrowing; superficial ulceration frequently causes bleeding. Characteristically, they are well differentiated. Local extension to the serosa and metastases in regional lymph nodes occur relatively early, whereas blood spread, mainly to the liver, is usually late. The overall 5-year survival is about 50%, but staging at the time of surgical resection (Chapter 10) is important—with tumours confined to the bowel wall it exceeds 85%, whereas when hepatic metastases are present it is less than 5%.

PERITONEUM

Normal

The peritoneal cavity is a potential space between the parietal peritoneum (lining the abdominal wall) and the visceral peritoneum (covering the enclosed viscera). Its free surfaces bear a flattened mesothelial cell lining and contain numerous macrophages.

Inflammation

Inflammation may be acute or chronic, localised or generalised.

Acute peritonitis is often secondary either to direct spread from an adjacent acute inflammatory focus (e.g. appendicitis, diverticulitis, pancreatitis and cholecystitis) or to gastrointestinal tract perforation (e.g. in peptic ulceration, Crohn's disease, ulcerative colitis and carcinoma). Acute inflammation develops, and often a copious acute inflammatory exudate is produced. It is a serious, potentially fatal condition requiring immediate active treatment and correction or removal of the underlying cause. Although resolution may occur, abscesses and fibrous scar tissue formation often develop; the latter may subsequently cause intestinal obstruction.

Chronic peritonitis, formerly commonly due to tuberculosis, is now uncommon. The major complication is intestinal obstruction due to excessive fibrosis.

Ascites

Ascites is excess intraperitoneal fluid. It may be encountered in generalised oedema states (e.g. cardiac failure and the nephrotic syndrome—Chapter 8) and in chronic liver diseases associated with portal hypertension (Chapter 17). Under these circumstances, it is usually sterile, but secondary bacterial infection is not uncommon. Excess intraperitoneal fluid is invariably a feature of the inflammatory exudate in acute peritonitis (see above).

Tumours

Primary neoplasms, both benign and malignant, are very rare. In contrast, secondary tumours are common, particularly from gastric, pancreatic, colonic and ovarian carcinomata; they are often numerous and extensive (carcinomatosis peritonei).

DENTAL ASPECTS

A few alimentary tract diseases can affect the oral mucosa or may occur as part of a syndrome with other abnormalities of the jaw bones or overlying soft tissues. Occasionally, dental practitioners may be the first to suspect intestinal disease.

Coeliac disease. There is a markedly increased incidence of coeliac disease in patients with oral aphthous ulceration (discussed in Chapter 15).

Ulcerative colitis. The commonest oral mucosal manifestation of ulcerative colitis is aphthous ulceration.

Crohn's disease. In addition to aphthous ulceration, oral presentation of Crohn's disease includes linear, fissuring ulceration and irregular swelling of the lips and cheeks to produce a 'cobblestone' appearance. Sometimes, oral lesions precede intestinal symptoms. Microscopically, the features are similar to those elsewhere, namely granulomatous inflammation and a chronically inflamed, oedematous fibroconnective tissue.

Peutz–Jeghers syndrome. As the associated intestinal polyps are often asymptomatic, pigmentation may well be the presenting feature.

Gardner's syndrome. The osteomas can be recognised radiologically as radiodense masses, and therefore this syndrome may be suspected on routine dental radiography.

17

Hepatic, biliary and pancreatic diseases

Liver
Normal
Circulatory disorders
Hepatocellular necrosis
Hepatitis
Cirrhosis
Liver failure
Portal hypertension

Tumours
Jaundice
Gallbladder and biliary tract
Normal
Inflammation
Calculi
Duct obstruction
Tumours

Pancreas
Normal
Inflammation
Fibrocystic disease (mucoviscidosis)
Diabetes mellitus
Tumours
Dental aspects

LIVER

Normal

The basic architectural unit is the *lobule*. At the centre of each lobule is a hepatic vein tributary (the *central vein*); at the periphery are several *portal tracts* comprising branches of hepatic artery, portal vein, bile ducts and lymphatics embedded in fibrous tissue. Within the lobules are narrow columns of liver cells (*hepatocytes*) arranged radially from central vein to portal tracts; the columns are separated by *sinusoids* (lined by vascular endothelium and phagocytic Kupffer cells, and conveying blood from hepatic arteries and portal veins to the central vein) and intralobular *bile canaliculi* (draining bile into portal tract bile ducts).

The liver has numerous physiological functions, including metabolism and storage (proteins, carbohydrates, fats and vitamins), synthesis (plasma proteins and enzymes) and detoxication (many endogenous waste products and exogenous toxins). Most drugs are metabolised by the liver.

Many liver abnormalities are interrelated and overlap. In addition, individual abnormalities have several causes, and each causative agent may produce different structural changes.

Circulatory disorders

The hepatic artery and portal vein provide a dual blood supply which is mixed within sinusoids; *infarction*, therefore, is uncommon. Centrilobular hepatocytes are furthest away from the portal tract branches of these vessels and are therefore most susceptible to hypoxic and ischaemic damage.

Chronic passive venous congestion. This is due to chronic right ventricular cardiac failure (Chapter 13). Hepatic venous pressure, and hence intralobular central venous pressure, is raised, producing sinusoidal dilatation and congestion with chronic hypoxia of centrilobular hepatocytes. These liver cells undergo degeneration, fatty change and, ultimately, necrosis; in contrast, peripheral (i.e. periportal) hepatocytes remain relatively normal. At this stage, the liver presents a very characteristic mottled macroscopic appearance of alternating congestion and pallor resembling a nutmeg—hence 'nutmeg liver'. Later, with more extensive centrilobular necrosis, progressive replacement by fibrous tissue occurs and cirrhosis may ultimately develop.

Shock liver. Shock (Chapter 8) may cause acute ischaemic centrilobular necrosis and liver function disturbances (see below).

Hepatocellular necrosis

Hepatocellular necrosis, to some extent, is common in liver diseases, and may be focal, confluent or massive; there is usually an associated acute and/or chronic inflammatory cell infiltrate.

Focal necrosis involves small groups of liver cells, the distribution of which is random and unrelated to basic lobular architecture. Causes include bacterial toxaemia, viral hepatitis and drug-induced damage. Regeneration usually occurs, and hepatic function is rarely impaired significantly.

Confluent necrosis affects larger groups of cells, and is often related to lobule zones. Centrilobular necrosis is seen in circulatory disorders (with anoxia and ischaemia—see above), viral hepatitis and with specific toxins (e.g. paracetamol, chloroform and carbon tetrachloride); midzonal necrosis is characteristic of yellow fever; peripheral (periportal) necrosis is produced by phosphorous poisoning. Occasionally (e.g. in viral hepatitis), confluent necrosis extends across lobular zones to produce *bridging necrosis*. Liver function impairment is proportional to the extent of hepatocellular necrosis. Results are very variable—if the cause is removed, regeneration will occur, particularly if the basic architectural connective tissue framework remains intact; if this framework is focally disrupted, areas of fibrosis (*postnecrotic scarring*) appear; if the cause persists, cirrhosis may ultimately develop; finally, progression to massive necrosis may occur.

Massive necrosis involves almost all hepatocytes. The usual causes are viral hepatitis and specific toxins (as in confluent necrosis above). Death from liver failure invariably results.

Hepatitis

Hepatitis is diffuse hepatic inflammation. It may be acute or chronic, although some overlap is common, and due to viruses, drugs, autoimmune disease, alcohol, biliary diseases or metabolic disorders; the last three are considered later with cirrhosis.

Acute

Acute hepatitis is usually viral, and two main types, A and B, are described.

Type A (infectious) hepatitis. The virus is invariably transmitted via the faecal–oral route; it has an incubation period of 2–6 weeks and occurs most commonly in children. Only one serotype exists, and immunity is produced by specific antibodies. Clinical symptoms are mild, and many cases are asymptomatic.

Type B (serum) hepatitis. The virus is usually transmitted by intravascular inoculation (e.g. in intravenous drug addiction, tattooing and in renal dialysis units); sexual transmission is also possible. It has an incubation period of 2–6 months and occurs at any age. Overall, clinical symptoms are more severe than in type A, and mortality in the acute episode is much higher. The virus consists of two components—a central infective core (Dane particle) and an outer surface envelope. These components possess separate and distinct antigenic determinants—hepatitis B core antigen (*HBcAg*) and hepatitis B surface antigen (*HBsAg*); the latter is also known as the Australia antigen following its initial discovery in an Aborigine. Other serological subtypes exist, the most important being the 'e' antigen (*HBeAg*), a breakdown product of HBcAg; its presence is related to Dane particle formation, and its persistence is associated with infectivity. Following primary infection, antibodies to these different antigens are produced. Anti-HBcAg antibodies (HBcAb) develop quickly; production of antibodies to HBsAg (HBsAb) is delayed, but once developed they persist and are considered protective; subsequently, their presence indicates past infection. Host immunological responses determine clinical outcome—most patients eradicate the virus completely; a few develop chronic hepatitis which may progress to cirrhosis; a few become asymptomatic chronic carriers. In this country, the incidence of HBsAg in blood donors is about 1:800; of these, 82% have antibodies to HBeAg (HBeAb) and are therefore up to one million times less likely to transmit the disease than the remaining 18% who are HBeAg positive but lack HBeAb. The carrier rate in the United Kingdom is therefore less than 0.1% of the total population; in parts of the Far East and Africa, however, it approaches 20%. Individuals with a significantly higher risk of carrying the disease include intravenous drug addicts, homosexuals, institutionalised people (e.g. prisoners and the mentally subnormal) and those with a history of liver disease.

Other. Other *viruses* may occasionally cause acute hepatitis, including herpes simplex, rubella and Epstein–Barr. Recently, *non-A:non-B hepatitis* (i.e. due to neither hepatitis A nor hepatitis B virus) has been described following blood transfusions; the causative agent(s) remain unknown, but asymptomatic chronic carriers must obviously exist.

Pathology. In most cases, there is focal liver cell necrosis; occasionally it is confluent; rarely it is massive (above). Factors determining extent and type of necrosis are unknown.

Chronic

Chronic hepatitis indicates continuous chronic hepatic inflammation for at least 6 months. It may be seen under three circumstances—in some patients, predominantly males, it is due to persistent hepatitis B virus; in some, 80% of whom are female, it is an autoimmune disease (sometimes designated *lupoid hepatitis*); in some it represents a reaction to drugs, particularly methyldopa and isoniazid. Two histological types are described.

Chronic persistent hepatitis. This indicates that the chronic inflammatory cell infiltrate is confined to portal tracts and does not extend into liver lobules. Clinical symptoms are usually mild, and ultimately resolution may occur; progression to cirrhosis does not develop.

Chronic aggressive (chronic active) hepatitis. In addition to chronic inflammatory cells within portal tracts, there is extension into adjacent peripheral (periportal) lobular zones with associated liver cell degeneration and necrosis ('piecemeal necrosis'). Portal and periportal fibrosis occurs, and this, together with hepatocellular regeneration, leads ultimately to cirrhosis in most cases. In addition, features of acute hepatitis may be present, and foci of more extensive, confluent necrosis may be seen. Clinical symptoms are usually more severe than with chronic persistent hepatitis, and when the autoimmune disease is responsible, other abnormalities (e.g. skin rashes and arthritis) may be present.

Cirrhosis

Cirrhosis is an irreversible, generalised liver disease where the lobular architecture is completely disorganised by nodules of regenerated liver cells and diffuse fibrous bands; it follows prolonged hepatocellular necrosis with continuing chronic inflammation and progressive replacement fibrosis. As regeneration and fibrosis progress the intrahepatic circulation is distorted and compressed, the resulting ischaemia contributing further to hepatocellular necrosis.

Macroscopic features

Cirrhotic livers are usually smaller than normal. The regeneration nodules are visible both externally and on section; they may all be small and approximately the same size (*micronodular cirrhosis*), or larger and more irregular (*macronodular cirrhosis*). Nodule size is sometimes used for classification, but is of limited value as many cases show features of both (*mixed cirrhosis*).

Aetiology

Aetiology provides the best classification, although, in this country, the cause remains unknown in almost 50% of cases.

Cryptogenic cirrhosis indicates unknown aetiology (i.e. idiopathic).

Alcoholic cirrhosis accounts for about 25% of cases. Alcohol is directly toxic to hepatocytes, and produces several lesions related to quantity and duration of alcohol excess. The earliest manifestation is fat accumulation within hepatocytes (*fatty change*); this is reversible, and does not by itself progress to cirrhosis. However, with prolonged abuse, predominantly centrilobular *alcoholic hepatitis* (focal hepatocellular necrosis with polymorph infiltration) and associated *hepatic fibrosis* appear in about one-third of patients at risk; in about one-third of these, continued alcohol excess causes relatively slow progression to a mainly micronodular cirrhosis. Factors involved in development of alcoholic hepatitis and cirrhosis are largely unknown, but only about 10% of alcoholics develop cirrhosis.

Posthepatitic cirrhosis is responsible for almost 20% of cases. It is usually macronodular, and develops in patients with chronic hepatitis (see above).

Primary biliary cirrhosis is an uncommon autoimmune disease with immunologically mediated intrahepatic bile duct destruction. It develops in middle age, and is much commoner in women (F:M about 9:1). Initial features are of obstructive jaundice (see below), but a mainly micronodular cirrhosis ultimately develops.

Secondary biliary cirrhosis appears with prolonged, unrelieved biliary outflow obstruction (see below). Bile accumulation within the liver (*cholestasis*) is toxic to liver cells, causing necrosis, inflammation and, ultimately, cirrhosis.

Cirrhosis due to inborn errors of metabolism is rare. Causes include *haemochromatosis* (excess accumulation of iron—Chapter 7) and *Wilson's disease* (excess copper).

Results

Cirrhosis is progressive and untreatable, and invariably results in death sooner or later. It causes both liver failure and portal hypertension, and about 10% develop hepatocellular carcinoma (see below).

Liver failure

Liver failure is inadequate hepatocellular function. Its onset may be acute (with massive hepatocellular necrosis) or chronic (usually due to cirrhosis). As liver functions are multiple and complex, so liver failure is variable and involves many systems.

Jaundice represents inadequate excretion of bilirubin (see below). It is related to hepatocellular injury, but in cirrhosis there may also be some intrahepatic biliary obstruction. In fulminating acute massive necrosis, death may supervene before jaundice is apparent clinically.

Neurological abnormalities include mental changes, flapping tremor of the limbs and coma, and are related to circulating nitrogenous metabolites, including ammonia, normally detoxified by the liver.

Plasma protein deficiencies reflect inadequate hepatic synthesis, and include albumin (which may lead to hypoalbuminaemia and oedema—Chapter 8) and coagulation factors (particularly prothrombin and fibrinogen—Chapter 20).

Endocrine disturbances are mainly due to inadequate hepatic metabolism and inactivation of sex hormones. There is infertility, loss of body hair, mottling of palmar skin ('*liver palms*') and cutaneous capillary malformations ('*spider naevi*')

in both sexes; males may also show testicular atrophy and breast enlargement (*gynaecomastia*), whilst women may develop breast atrophy and menstrual irregularities.

Other features include low grade fever and a characteristic sweet smell to the breath (*foetor hepaticus*).

Portal hypertension

Portal hypertension, a rise in hydrostatic pressure within portal veins, is due to progressive compression and obstruction of intrahepatic portal venous radicles by hepatocellular regeneration and fibrosis. The major effect is to produce prominent anastomotic channels between portal and systemic venous systems, especially in and around the lower oesophagus (*oesophageal varices*—Chapter 16), rectum and umbilicus; mild, severe or even fatal haemorrhage from these channels is common. It also causes splenic enlargement (*splenomegaly*) and ascites.

Tumours

Benign

Benign tumours are rare, and include *adenomas* and cavernous *haemangiomas*. They are usually asymptomatic, although haemorrhage may occur.

Primary malignant

Primary malignant tumours account for only about 1% of malignancies in this country, but are several times more common in parts of Africa and Asia.

Hepatocellular carcinoma (*malignant hepatoma*) is the commonest, and over 75% develop in livers with established, usually macronodular cirrhosis, often due to hepatitis B virus. It may be a large, single infiltrating mass, but cases with multiple, smaller, discrete tumour nodules (presumably representing multifocal development) are fairly common. Intrahepatic local spread is often extensive, but extrahepatic lymphatic and haematogenous metastases are relatively infrequent. Prognosis is extremely poor—most patients are dead within 6 months.

Cholangiocarcinoma is much less common, but has an equally poor prognosis. It is derived from intrahepatic bile ducts and is usually unassociated with cirrhosis.

Haemangioendothelioma is very rare, but is of interest because of an association with industrial exposure to vinyl chloride monomer.

Secondary

Secondary tumours are very common, both from the alimentary tract via the portal vein and from elsewhere (particularly breast and bronchus) via the systemic circulation. Usually, multiple nodules, some of which may be quite large, are scattered throughout the liver.

Jaundice

Jaundice, although sometimes due to non-hepatic diseases, is considered here with liver disorders for convenience. It reflects excess bilirubin within the body, and causes yellowish skin discoloration. Normally, about 300 mg of bilirubin is produced daily, mostly from haemoglobin of effete red blood cells destroyed by the mononuclear phago- cyte (reticulo-endothelial) system. From there, it enters the circulation (bound to albumin as water- insoluble *unconjugated bilirubin*) to be taken up by liver cells, conjugated with glucuronic acid to form water-soluble *conjugated bilirubin* and excreted into bile; in the intestines, it is converted into *ster- cobilinogen*, some of which is absorbed to re-enter the liver (*the entero-hepatic circulation*) and a small quantity of which is excreted in the urine as *urobilinogen*. Three types are described, but some overlap is possible.

Haemolytic (prehepatic) jaundice reflects increased bilirubin production, and is due to increased red cell destruction (haemolysis—Chapter 20). The excess bilirubin is unconjugated, bound to albumin and water insoluble; it therefore does not appear in the urine (hence *acholuric jaundice*).

Hepatocellular (hepatic) jaundice is due to liver cell damage, and is seen with confluent or massive hepatocellular necrosis and cirrhosis. The excess bilirubin is usually a mixture of unconjugated and conjugated, and some therefore appears in the urine.

Obstructive (posthepatic) jaundice is usually caused by bile duct obstruction (see below); occasionally, an identical picture is seen with intrahepatic cholestasis due to idiosyncratic drug reactions (e.g. to chlorpromazine) and rarely to primary biliary cirrhosis. The excess bilirubin is mainly conjugated, and the urine is therefore dark in colour. As little or no bile enters the intestines, stercobilinogen is largely absent, and the faeces are pale.

GALLBLADDER AND BILIARY TRACT

Normal

The *gallbladder* is a pear-shaped sac lying on the undersurface of the liver. It is about 10 cm in length and up to 3 cm in maximum diameter, and has a capacity of 30–50 ml. It is lined by mucus- secreting tall columnar epithelium arranged in narrow rugae. The gallbladder stores bile from the liver and concentrates it tenfold by absorbing water and electrolytes. When food enters the proximal duodenum, bile is discharged along the common bile duct and into the distal duodenum, gallbladder contraction being stimulated hor- monally by cholecystokinin.

The *biliary tract* comprises common hepatic, cystic and common bile ducts. The *common hepatic duct* is formed from the right and left hepatic ducts soon after they emerge from the liver. The *cystic duct* joins the common hepatic duct to the gallbladder. The *common bile duct*, formed by the junction of cystic and common hepatic ducts, passes down, through the head of the pancreas, into the duodenum.

Bile comprises bile pigments (mainly bilirubin), bile acids and salts (to emulsify fat in the intes- tines and to facilitate absorption of fat-soluble vitamins and calcium), cholesterol and mucin. Some drugs and poisons are also excreted in bile.

Inflammation

Cholecystitis may be acute or chronic.

Acute cholecystitis invariably follows cystic duct obstruction by calculi (below). Initially, about 90% are sterile, and the inflammation is probably chemically induced, but secondary bacterial infection usually soon develops, and about 80% are infected by the fourth day; the organisms are often colonic bacteria, and although the route whereby they reach the gallbladder is unknown, lymphatics are usually suggested. The resulting acute inflammation is variable, but often severe, with intraluminal pus (*empyema of the gallbladder*), mucosal ulceration, mural abscesses and necrosis, and serosal fibrin deposition. The most important complication is perforation followed by peritonitis.

Chronic cholecystitis may follow acute cholecystitis, but usually arises de novo, and calculi are present in over 90% of cases. Bacteria are usually absent, and the chronic inflammation is probably induced chemically. The gallbladder is contracted, the wall is thickened by hypertrophic muscle and fibrous tissue, and the mucosa is flattened and atrophic. Histologically, focal, transmural chronic inflammation is also been, and epithelium often extends down into the muscle coat to form *Aschoff-Rokitansky sinuses*. Resolution is uncommon, and the usual treatment is surgical removal (*cholecystectomy*).

Calculi

Calculi (*gallstones*) are present in almost 10% of adults. They are usually found in the middle aged and elderly, particularly multiparous and obese females (F:M about 4:1). Gallstones represent precipitated bile, and are almost always formed in the gallbladder.

Aetiology. The major factor is alteration in bile composition, particularly the cholesterol:bile acid and phospholipid ratio—a relative excess of cholesterol promotes stone formation. Reasons for these changes are unknown, but local stasis and mild infection may contribute.

Types. About 90% are *mixed*, composed mainly of cholesterol, with bile pigments, calcium salts and a protein matrix; they are invariably multiple, irregular in shape (usually smooth and multifaceted) and of very variable size. The remaining 10% are *pure*—some contain cholesterol (usually solitary, large, round or oval and yellow); some are *pigment stones* of calcium bilirubinate (multiple, black, small and irregular in shape), and associated with prolonged increased haemolysis (Chapter 20); rarely, they consist of calcium carbonate.

Results. Many remain within the gallbladder (*cholelithiasis*) and produce no symptoms (silent stones). They may, however, predispose to inflammation (both acute and chronic cholecystitis) and cause cystic duct or common bile duct obstruction; they are associated with acute pancreatitis (see below). Very rarely, chronic irritation may lead to neoplasia.

Duct obstruction

Duct obstruction may be partial or total, and is occasionally intermittent.

Causes

Causes are numerous, and may be intraluminal, intramural or extramural.

Intraluminal causes are usually calculi; occasionally, there may be failure of normal embryological development (*biliary atresia*), and fibrocystic disease is sometimes responsible.

Intramural causes include congenital, post-inflammatory or post-traumatic fibrous strictures and tumours.

Extramural compression is seen with carcinomas of pancreatic head, ampulla of Vater and duodenum, primary or metastatic tumours in lymph nodes around the porta hepatis, chronic pancreatitis and, rarely, accidental ligation during abdominal operations.

Effects

Significant obstruction produces obstructive jaundice and predisposes to local infection (*ascending cholangitis*). When prolonged, secondary biliary cirrhosis may develop.

Tumours

Tumours of the gallbladder and bile ducts together account for approximately 1.5% of all malignancies. Benign tumours in both sites are very rare.

Gallbladder carcinoma is associated with gallstones in almost 90% of cases, and is therefore more common in women; it is usually an adenocarcinoma. Local invasion of liver and bile ducts (often causing jaundice) occurs early, as does lymphatic and haematogenous spread; prognosis is thus poor.

Extrahepatic bile duct carcinoma is less frequently associated with gallstones, and is, overall, slightly commoner in men. It is an adenocarcinoma, and most often arises in the common bile duct. It usually grows fairly slowly, and invariably presents with progressive obstructive jaundice.

PANCREAS

Normal

The pancreas lies transversely across the posterior abdominal wall behind the stomach. It comprises head (through which the common bile duct passes), body and tail. Structurally, it consists of two separate, unrelated components—*exocrine* (lobular, glandular acini secreting enzymes, mainly trypsin, chymotrypsin, amylase and lipase, for intestinal digestion) and *endocrine* (islets of Langerhans secreting several hormones, particularly insulin and glucagon, directly into the circulation).

Inflammation

Pancreatitis may be acute or chronic.

Acute pancreatitis

This is acute haemorrhagic necrosis due to local release of pancreatic enzymes. It is fairly common, more so in females than males, and usually develops in middle-aged or elderly patients. It is initially sterile, but secondary bacterial infection often occurs.

Aetiology. Several predisposing factors exist, mainly gallstones, chronic alcoholism and shock with hypotension; less common ones include trauma (both blunt and penetrating injuries), hypothermia, mumps and pancreatic duct obstruction. Mechanisms whereby necrosis is initiated, however, remain largely unknown.

Pathology. The gland is usually swollen and firm, with areas of haemorrhage and necrosis.

Microscopy reveals coagulative acinar necrosis, blood vessel necrosis producing haemorrhage, fat necrosis (from liberated lipase) and variable, usually mild polymorph infiltration. Peritoneal involvement is common, with accumulation of blood-stained serous fluid and multiple foci of fat necrosis.

Clinical features. Presentation is usually intense abdominal pain, vomiting and shock. Pancreatic enzymes enter the circulation, and measurements of serum and urine amylase levels represent important diagnostic tests.

Results. In severe cases, mortality is high. In less severe cases, complete resolution is uncommon and healing by fibrosis, often with cyst formation, usually occurs. Recurrent attacks are frequent; progression to chronic pancreatitis is rare.

Chronic pancreatitis

This usually arises de novo, and is uncommon. The major association is with chronic alcoholism; a few have haemochromatosis (Chapter 7). The gland is firm and shrunken, often with focal calcification and cyst formation. Histologically, there is progressive fibrous replacement of acinar tissue and mild chronic inflammation; initially, islets of Langerhans are spared, but they too are ultimately replaced by fibrosis to produce diabetes mellitus. Clinical features, when present, may also include intermittent or continuous abdominal pain, malabsorption (Chapter 16) and obstructive jaundice.

Fibrocystic disease

Fibrocystic disease (mucoviscidosis) affects exocrine mucous gland secretions, chiefly in pancreas and respiratory, alimentary and biliary tracts; the mucus is abnormally thick and viscid. It is usually inherited as an autosomal recessive, and affects about 1 in every 2000 infants in this country. Aetiology is unknown, but some underlying enzymatic or metabolic disorder is probably responsible. In the pancreas, abnormal mucus obstructs ducts, producing progressive acinar replacement by fibrosis; malabsorption usually develops, but diabetes mellitus is uncommon. Elsewhere, pulmonary involvement predisposes to infections and fibrosis; alimentary symptoms are usually obstruction, possibly with perforation; biliary complications are obstruction and secondary biliary cirrhosis. In affected patients, sweat contains excess sodium and chloride—a useful diagnostic test. Prognosis, although somewhat variable, is poor—very few patients survive childhood.

Diabetes mellitus

Diabetes mellitus is a metabolic disorder due to absolute or relative insulin deficiency with consequent elevated blood sugar levels (*hyperglycaemia*). It is common, affecting, to some extent, almost 1% of the population in this country, and may be primary or secondary.

Primary

Primary diabetes is of unknown aetiology. Two types are described, and in both, pancreatic islet morphology is often remarkably normal.

Type I (juvenile, early-onset or insulin-dependent diabetes) may show a familial tendency, and auto-antibodies may be present. It usually develops in childhood or early adult life, and insulin is required for treatment. Onset shows definite seasonal variation, and viral infection may be a precipitating factor.

Type II (maturity, late-onset or non-insulin-dependent diabetes) develops insidiously, particularly in elderly, obese females. Dietary control, with or without oral hypoglycaemic drugs, is usually sufficient for treatment.

Secondary

Secondary diabetes is due either to destructive pancreatic disease (e.g. chronic pancreatitis and haemochromatosis) or to excess insulin antagonists (e.g. growth hormone and glucocorticosteroids—Chapter 19).

Complications

These are mainly vascular and infective.

Vascular. Larger arteries show atheroma earlier, more severely and more extensively than in non-diabetics; all atheroma complications are therefore common in diabetics (Chapter 12). Smaller arteries, arterioles and capillaries show abnormal basement membrane thickening by amorphous, acellular, eosinophilic material and endothelial proliferation (*diabetic microangiopathy* or *diabetic hyalinisation*): this produces glomerular sclerosis (Chapter 18), retinal changes (diabetic retinopathy) and ischaemic peripheral nerve damage (diabetic neuropathy).

Infections. Diabetics have increased susceptibility to almost all infections (Chapter 5), especially in skin, lungs and urinary tract.

Prognosis

With insulin treatment, death in hyperglycaemic coma is rare; however, life expectancy is reduced, mainly by accelerated atheroma and glomerular disease.

Tumours

Benign exocrine tumours are rare.

Adenocarcinoma is derived from exocrine glands. It is fairly common, accounting for almost 4% of all malignancies, and its incidence is increasing. It usually develops between 50 and 65 years of age; it is about twice as common in men, and almost twice as common in diabetics. Most (about 60%) arise in the pancreatic head, and invariably present with progressive, often painless obstructive jaundice; tumours in the body (25%) and tail (15%) are usually clinically silent until well established. Spread—direct, lymphatic, haematogenous and peritoneal—occurs early, and prognosis is very poor.

Islet cell tumours of endocrine origin are much less common, and arise in younger patients (usually 30–50 years of age). About 90% are benign, but it is impossible to predict, on histological grounds, which will metastasise. Almost 20% are small and multiple, and may be associated with adenomas in other endocrine organs. About 60% secrete one or more hormones, including insulin (causing multiple episodes of hypoglycaemia) and gastrin (producing gastric acid hypersecretion and intractable chronic peptic ulceration).

DENTAL ASPECTS

Type B (*serum*) *hepatitis* presents an important risk to all health care personnel, as only 0.0001 ml of blood containing HBeAg is required to transmit the disease. Unfortunately, carriers exist (see above); most appear healthy and are asymptomatic, and only a small proportion will have had overt clinical liver disease in the past. The blood of carriers who are HBsAg and HBeAg positive has high infectivity, but if antibodies against HBeAg (HBeAb) are present, the risk to other patients and staff is very greatly reduced. Even so, it is wise to take extra precautions concerning the sterilisation of hand pieces and instruments, the type of impression materials used, and to wear gloves, masks and spectacles. Should the dentist be innoculated accidentally with blood from a carrier, an injection of hepatitis B immune globulin will reduce greatly the risk of developing the disease: this presupposes that the dentist is 'at risk',—that is, is not a carrier and has no circulating antibodies against the disease. It is recommended that staff be vaccinated routinely against hepatitis B infection.

18

Urinary tract diseases

Kidneys
Normal
Congenital abnormalities
Pyelonephritis
Glomerular diseases
Hypertension

Hydronephrosis
Renal calculi
Acute tubular necrosis
Renal failure
Renal transplantation
Tumours

Ureters
Bladder
Normal
Inflammation
Tumours

Urethra
Normal
Inflammation
Obstruction
Dental aspects

KIDNEYS

Normal

Kidneys filter numerous waste products from the plasma and maintain normal body electrolyte, fluid and acid–base levels. These functions are performed by the *nephrons*, approximately one million of which are found in each kidney. One nephron comprises a *glomerulus* (a mass of capillaries, confined within Bowman's capsule, through which the plasma is initially filtered) and a long *tubule* (different segments of which have different functions and names—proximal convoluted tubule, loop of Henle, distal convoluted tubule and collecting tubule), which modifies considerably the glomerular filtrate, mainy by active absorption, until it finally emerges as *urine*. All glomeruli and convoluted tubules lie within the *renal cortex*; the *medulla* contains loops of Henle and collecting tubules, and projects between the *calyces* and into the *renal pelvis* as *papillae*.

Congenital abnormalities

As embryological renal development and migration are very complex, minor unimportant abnormalities are not uncommon—persistent fetal lobulation, simple cortical cysts, abnormal location (e.g. at pelvic brim or within pelvis) and partial fusion, usually at the lower poles (*horseshoe kidney*). A few minor anomalies (e.g. aberrant renal arteries and double pelvis and ureter) may cause obstruction and hydronephrosis (below). Occasionally, one or both kidneys may fail to develop (*renal agenesis*); absence of both rapidly proves fatal.

Polycystic disease is an hereditary condition where both kidneys are gradually replaced by numerous cysts until the intervening normal renal tissue is destroyed. Renal function is progressively impaired, and renal failure ultimately develops. Although congenital, it usually presents in early or middle adult life, and is inherited as an autosomal dominant.

Pyelonephritis

Pyelonephritis is literally inflammation of renal pelvis and renal parenchyma. It may be acute or chronic, unilateral or bilateral, focal or diffuse. Usually, the bacteria responsible reach the kidney via the urinary tract (i.e. they are *ascending infections*); less commonly, organisms arrive in the blood in septicaemia or pyaemia and produce multiple abscesses. The major predisposing factor in ascending infections is partial urinary tract obstruction, and hence some hydronephrosis may be present also. Obstruction promotes urinary stasis (which provides a good bacterial culture medium) and urinary reflux during micturition; it may be due to major or minor congenital abnormalities, pressure from an enlarged, pregnant uterus, uterine prolapse or prostatic hyperplasia (see below). All ascending infections are much more common in females, probably because it is easier for organisms to enter the bladder along their much shorter urethras; the bacteria responsible are usually faecal in origin, the commonest being *Escherichia coli*.

Acute

Acute pyelonephritis is typical acute inflammation with considerable local tissue destruction and abscess formation. Histologically, the polymorph infiltration is mainly within and around renal tubules and the pelvic epithelium; numerous polymorphs, together with the causative bacteria, are present in the urine. With early, appropriate antibiotic treatment, considerable resolution will occur, but some healing by fibrosis is common; recurrent acute attacks are fairly frequent, and progression to chronic pyelonephritis may develop.

Chronic

Chronic pyelonephritis may vary from mild and focal to severe, diffuse and bilateral. Its aetiology is often uncertain; it may follow multiple, recurrent episodes of acute pyelonephritis, but usually no such history exists, and it may represent prolonged, low grade, subclinical infection. With extensive disease, the kidney is smaller than normal, and the cortex shows numerous, irregular, depressed scars; the pelvis and calyces are distorted and often somewhat dilated. Histologically, there is prominent interstitial chronic inflammation and fibrosis with associated glomerular and tubular destruction; many residual tubules are dilated and contain protein casts, and smaller vessels often show prominent hypertensive changes. Mild focal chronic pyelonephritis is usually asymptomatic and, although progression is possible, is a relatively unimportant incidental finding; severe, extensive, bilateral disease, however, is very important as a cause of secondary hypertension, renal function impairment and, ultimately, renal failure.

Tuberculosis

Renal involvement follows haematogenous spread, usually from a primary or secondary pulmonary focus, and may represent miliary tuberculosis or single organ disease. The latter, which is now relatively uncommon, is seen as numerous caseating tubercles which gradually enlarge and combine until extensive destruction results.

Glomerular diseases

Glomerular diseases are conditions with significant glomerular involvement; they may be primary, or secondary to multisystem diseases.

Primary

Primary glomerular diseases constitute the group where glomeruli are the sole target for the disease processes. They are often referred to collectively as *glomerulonephritis*, an unfortunate term as true glomerular inflammation is rare and the changes elsewhere in the kidney are secondary. Following the widespread and routine use of renal biopsy techniques, knowledge and understanding of glomerular pathology has expanded considerably in the past 20 years; numerous detailed and lengthy classifications exist, but only a few basic concepts are considered here.

Immunopathology. Two distinct immunological mechanisms are known. The more common is *immune complex disease*, a type III hypersensitivity reaction (Chapter 6), where circulating immune (antigen–antibody) complexes are deposited in glomeruli. The antibodies are those normally found in the circulation (i.e. IgG, IgM or IgA); the nature and source of the antigens remain unknown in most cases, although streptococci, neoplasms (usually malignant), drugs and specific infections are sometimes involved. Several factors determine whether circulating complexes deposit in glomeruli and, if so, where; the most important are physical size and molecular weight. The second, and much less common mechanism is *antiglomerular basement membrane antibody disease*, a type II hypersensitivity reaction with circulating antibodies (usually IgG) directed specifically against glomerular basement membrane antigenic determinants. Why these antibodies should suddenly appear is unknown. Often, there is some cross-reaction with pulmonary alveolar basement membranes producing variable intrapulmonary haemorrhage (*Goodpasture's syndrome*). Although only these two mechanisms are known, there remain some forms of glomerulonephritis due to other, as yet unknown processes.

Histopathology. All histopathological classifications are long and complex, but two main changes are seen—cellular proliferation and capillary basement membrane thickening; they vary in extent and severity, but tend to reflect the site and intensity of the causative immunopathology. Proliferation may be of one or more endogenous glomerular cells, or of the epithelial cells lining Bowman's capsules; the latter represents severe glomerular damage and presents as glomerular tuft compression by *crescents* (i.e. *crescentic glomerulonephritis*). Sometimes, proliferation is confined to only some glomeruli, the remainder being normal. Membrane thickening may be the only abnormality (*membranous glomerulonephritis*) or it may be associated with cellular proliferation. Occasionally, glomerular dysfunction is present with no significant glomerular structural abnormality ('*minimal change disease*').

Prognosis. Prognosis is very variable, but can, to some extent, be predicted by renal biopsy appearances. Some (e.g. minimal change disease) improve spontaneously, and, although they may recur, are associated with an excellent long term outlook; some (e.g. many cases of membranous glomerulonephritis) persist for many years without significant renal function deterioration; others (e.g. crescentic glomerulonephritis) progress, with function deterioration and secondary hypertension, into chronic renal failure. Antiglomerular basement membrane antibody disease is usually associated with severe glomerular changes (e.g. crescents) and has a poor prognosis.

Treatment. Unfortunately, with the exception of corticosteroid therapy in minimal change disease, no treatment successfully influences the natural course in primary glomerular diseases.

Secondary

Here, glomeruli are involved in multisystem diseases.

Diabetes mellitus. Some glomerular involvement is very common in long standing diabetes, and over 50% of juvenile diabetics ultimately develop significant renal function impairment. There is intraglomerular deposition of acellular, eosinophilic material similar to that seen in basement membranes elsewhere (Chapter 17); this is usually diffuse, but in addition, may be seen discrete, amorphous masses (*Kimmelstiel–Wilson nodules*).

Amyloid disease. Whether primary or secondary, this disease almost always affects glomeruli to some extent (Chapter 7). There is progressive amyloid deposition which gradually replaces glomerular constituents and produces renal function impairment with, ultimately, renal failure. Amyloid is also deposited in and around tubules and in smaller blood vessels.

Systemic lupus erythematosus (SLE). This is one of the autoimmune connective tissue diseases (Chapter 23). Glomerular involvement is virtually 100% and is due to circulating immune complex deposition; almost any of the histopathological changes discussed above may be seen, and as many SLE patients present with glomerular dysfunction this diagnosis should always be considered. Although SLE may be modified by corticosteroid therapy, long term prognosis is usually related to severity of glomerular involvement, and death in renal failure is fairly common.

Clinical features

Although many glomerular diseases (both primary and secondary) exist, presentation is usually limited either to abnormal filtration of protein and/or red blood cells into the urine or to features of renal function impairment. Hence, the nature and type of underlying glomerular disease cannot be predicted by the mode of presentation, and biopsy is necessary for definitive diagnosis. Some patients are asymptomatic at presentation—mild *proteinuria* and/or *microscopic haematuria* are detected by routine urine testing (e.g. for insurance purposes or before employment): some notice *macroscopic haematuria*; many have the *nephrotic syndrome* (heavy proteinuria, hypoalbuminaemia and oedema—Chapter 8); a few develop features of renal failure (see below) without any preceding urinary symptoms. Glomerular diseases may present at any age, although different forms may be more associated with particular ages (e.g. minimal change disease in childhood).

Hypertension

Hypertension both causes and is caused by renal

disease; it is discussed in detail in Chapter 12, and only briefly here. It is benign or malignant, essential (primary) or secondary.

Benign essential hypertension. Renal changes are largely due to ischaemia following arterial and arteriolar wall thickening and luminal narrowing. The cortex shows multiple, small, superficial, depressed scars presenting as subcapsular granularity, and there may be slight overall reduction in renal size. Histologically, occasional glomeruli are gradually replaced by acellular, hyaline material and associated tubules become atrophic. The changes are usually mild and focal; significant function impairment is uncommon, and renal failure is rare.

Malignant essential hypertension. This causes severe damage, and many patients die in renal failure, even with antihypertensive drug treatment. There is glomerular ischaemia due to the vascular changes, and some glomeruli often also show fibrinoid necrosis and intracapillary thrombosis.

Secondary hypertension. Whether benign or malignant, this is usually due to renal diseases; the major causes (chronic pyelonephritis, primary and secondary glomerular diseases, polycystic kidneys, hydronephrosis and some primary renal tumours) are discussed elsewhere in this chapter. Occasionally, it follows unilateral or bilateral renal artery stenosis, usually due to atheroma of either the renal arteries themselves or the aorta around their origins. When it is due to renal disease, a vicious circle becomes established—the already damaged kidney causes hypertension and hypertensive vascular disease, which in turn cause further renal damage.

Hydronephrosis

Hydronephrosis is dilatation of the renal pelvis and calyces due to progressive urinary tract obstruction, the site of which determines whether it is unilateral or bilateral, and whether other components (e.g. ureters and bladder) are also dilated.

Causes

Causes are intraluminal, intramural, extramural or neuromuscular, and may lie anywhere between the pelvi-ureteric junction and distal urethra.

Intraluminal causes are usually impacted calculi.

Intramural lesions include tumours, postinflammatory fibrous strictures (particularly urethral) and congenital abnormalities (valves and strictures).

Extramural compression may be from prostatic hyperplasia (see below), extrinsic tumours (e.g. of uterine cervix), pregnant uterus and aberrant renal vessels (usually around the pelvi-ureteric junction).

Neuromuscular dysfunction is seen in spinal cord diseases; occasionally, unilateral hydronephrosis occurs without any obvious structural cause, and neuromuscular incoordination is probably responsible.

Results

Significant hydronephrosis causes progressive parenchymal destruction, atrophy and fibrosis; in severe cases only a thin rim of renal tissue remains. Superadded secondary infection is common. Unilateral hydronephrosis does not impair renal function significantly, although secondary hypertension may result; bilateral hydronephrosis, if severe, will cause renal failure.

Renal calculi

Renal calculi represent precipitation of urinary salts around organic material. Their composition varies considerably, and they are often mixed. About 90% contain calcium (and hence are usually radio-opaque); in about two-thirds, it is combined with oxalate and in one-third with phosphate, often also with magnesium and/or ammonium. Approximately 5% comprise pure uric acid. Renal stones lie within the renal pelvis. They may be single or multiple, unilateral or bilateral; they are usually small, but may be large and branched, reflecting the shape of the pelvi-calyceal system ('*stag-horn*' calculi).

Causes. Several predisposing factors are known, but often none applies. Renal calculi are common in primary hyperparathyroidism, where excess calcium and phosphate are excreted in the urine (Chapter 19). Phosphates are less soluble in alkaline urine, and prolonged alkalinity (e.g. in some urine infections) promotes stone formation. Urinary stasis from obstruction also predisposes.

Effects. Calculi may cause obstruction (of the pelvi-ureteric junction, ureter or bladder to produce hydronephrosis) or chronic inflammation. Associated chronic irritation may induce squamous metaplasia of renal pelvic or bladder transitional epithelium with possible subsequent malignant change.

Acute tubular necrosis

Metabolically, renal tubular epithelium is extremely active, and is therefore particularly susceptible to anoxic and toxic damage—acute tubular necrosis. Anoxia is usually associated with shock (e.g. haemorrhage, trauma, burns and incompatible blood transfusion—Chapter 8); relevant chemical toxins include carbon tetrachloride, ethylene glycol (used as antifreeze) and compounds of mercury, arsenic and chromium. Macroscopically, the kidneys are swollen and pale. Histologically, glomeruli are normal, but tubules show mild dilatation and epithelial flattening, degeneration and necrosis, with intraluminal cellular debris and proteinaceous material. At this stage, if the damage is extensive, the urine volume is reduced considerably and acute renal failure develops (see below). If causative factors are removed or corrected, epithelial regeneration occurs, and total structural and functional normality is restored fairly quickly. Although the main causes are known, the mechanisms whereby tubular damage is produced are ill understood.

Renal failure

Renal failure, indicating inadequate renal function, may be acute or chronic.

Acute renal failure. The term reflects rapidity of onset. The commonest cause is acute tubular necrosis; others include severe crescentic glomerulonephritis and malignant hypertension. There is a reduction in urine volume (*oliguria*) or even no urine produced (*anuria*); a rapid rise in waste and toxic nitrogenous metabolites (e.g. urea and creatinine) in the blood; fluid retention, often with oedema and hypertension; acid–base disturbances, with hydrogen ion retention (*acidosis*); electrolyte imbalance, especially a raised serum potassium (*hyperkalaemia*). Without active treatment (e.g.

peritoneal or haemodialysis), death occurs within several days, often from cardiac arrhythmias due to hyperkalaemia.

Chronic renal failure. This develops gradually over a much longer period of time. In this country, major causes are: primary glomerular diseases (50%); chronic pyelonephritis (20%, with female:male ratio about 2:1); polycystic kidneys (10%); vascular diseases (5%); others, including diabetes mellitus, amyloid, systemic lupus erythematosus and bilateral hydronephrosis (15%). The usual features (cf. acute renal failure) include retention of nitrogenous metabolites (uraemia), acidosis, hyperkalaemia, increased urine volume (*polyuria*), hypertension (usually secondary) and phosphate retention, which causes a reduction in plasma calcium and stimulates parathyroid hormone secretion (*secondary hyperparathyroidism*—Chapter 19). Later, changes may be found in other organs, including fibrinous pericarditis, alimentary tract haemorrhages, ulceration and inflammation (*uraemic colitis* or *enterocolitis*), pulmonary oedema with alveolar exudates (*uraemic pneumonitis*) generalised immune suppression and severe anaemia (normochromic, normocytic—Chapter 20). Chronic renal failure is irreversible, and patient survival depends on active intervention with either long term dialysis or successful renal transplantation.

Renal transplantation

Renal transplantation is becoming more popular as a treatment for chronic renal failure, but obviously depends on availability of suitable kidneys. The graft is inserted outside the peritoneum in an iliac fossa; donor renal vessels are anastomosed to the recipient's iliac vessels, and donor ureter is implanted directly into the recipient's bladder.

Rejection. Although anoxia between the time of donor death and transplantation often leads to transient acute tubular necrosis, the major problem is both antibody- and cell-mediated immunological graft rejection (Chapter 6). Matching of tissue types and ABO blood groups increases overall graft survival. Humoral-mediated rejection causes predominantly arterial damage (endothelial, intimal and medial proliferation and fibrinoid necrosis) with subsequent ischaemia; cellular rejection produces interstitial inflammation, oedema and tubular necrosis.

Treatment. Without immunosuppression by corticosteroid and cytotoxic drugs, rejection is rapid and complete; with treatment, it is delayed and often adequately controlled. Unfortunately, currently available drugs are non-specific, and suppress all immunological and inflammatory responses; consequently, transplant recipients show increased susceptibility to infection, particularly opportunistic (e.g. cytomegalovirus).

Tumours

Renal tumours may be benign or malignant, and if malignant, primary or secondary.

Benign tumours

The commonest is the *adenoma*, originating from tubular epithelium. It is invariably in the cortex and usually subcapsular. Few of these tumours exceed 1 cm in diameter, and almost all are asymptomatic and incidental findings; they are important only because they may develop into *adenocarcinomas* (see below). Rarely, benign tumours may arise from the renal connective tissue framework; the commonest is the medullary *fibroma*.

Primary malignant tumours

Primary malignant tumours account for approximately 1.5% of all malignancies in this country.

Adenocarcinoma, derived from renal tubular epithelium and originating in a pre-existing adenoma, is the commonest. It used to be called *hypernephroma*, as it was originally thought to arise from adrenal tissue incorporated into the kidney during embryological development. Although it may arise at virtually any age, its maximum incidence is between 50 and 60 years, and it is about twice as common in men. It is seen as expanding, solid cortical mass, often golden yellow in colour with areas of haemorrhage and necrosis. Microscopically it shows variable differentiation, but characteristically comprises large clear or granular cells containing lipid and glycogen. Clinically, about 60% present with painless haematuria and

about 50% have flank pain; only about 15% display the 'classical triad' of haematuria, loin pain and a palpable mass on clinical examination. Sometimes, the diagnosis is made only after investigation for such non-specific complaints as weight loss, unexplained fever and anaemia; a few present with symptoms from established metastases or abnormal hormonal production (e.g. *renin* causing hypertension and *erythropoietin* producing polycythaemia—Chapter 20). Usually, it grows slowly, and may be quite large at presentation, with local spread to adjacent structures (perinephric fat, colon, etc.): regional para-aortic lymph node metastases occur early—they are present in almost 25% of cases at initial operation. Haematogenous spread is also early, with venous involvement in about one-third of operation specimens; lungs are the commonest site for blood borne metastases—they may be large and solitary, and present radiologically as 'cannon-ball' lesions. Prognosis is influenced considerably by histological differentiation and extent of spread at presentation; overall 20–25% survive 10 years.

Nephroblastoma (Wilms' tumour) is rare, but as it usually occurs between 1 and 3 years of age, it is one of the commonest solid malignant tumours in infancy and early childhood. It arises in the renal cortex, and is derived from residual embryological tissues. Local, lymphatic and haematogenous spread occur early, but with vigorous radiotherapy and chemotherapy prognosis is now good.

Transitional cell carcinoma arises from pelvic epithelium. As these tumours are much more common in the bladder, they are discussed in this context below. In the kidney, they are usually poorly differentiated, and show extensive early local and lymphatic spread; although haematuria often occurs early, long term prognosis is poor.

Squamous cell carcinoma is a rare pelvic tumour. It is usually associated with calculi, and prognosis is extremely poor.

Secondary malignant tumours

These are not as common as might be expected from the large renal blood supply. Only about 5% of patients with disseminated carcinoma have renal metastases, and these are mainly from bronchus, breast and stomach. About 50% with disseminated lymphomas and leukaemias show renal involvement.

URETERS

Normal. Ureters are narrow, thick-walled tubes, lined by transitional epithelium, which convey urine from renal pelvis to bladder.

Pathology. One or both may be involved in more generalised urinary tract diseases.

Inflammation. This is due to ascending urinary tract infection and associated with *pyelonephritis* (see above) and/or *cystitis* (see below).

Hydroureter. This is dilatation due to lower urinary tract obstruction, and is discussed with *hydronephrosis* above.

Calculi. Occasionally, small calculi may become dislodged from the pelvis and enter the ureter. Transient passage down the ureter produces severe pain (renal colic); permanent impaction causes hydroureter and hydronephrosis.

Tumours. Almost always transitional cell in type, these are discussed below.

BLADDER

Normal

The urinary bladder is a distensible muscular sac, lined by transitional epithelium, in which urine is stored temporarily before being released, usually when convenient, to the outside world via the urethra. Urine in the bladder is normally sterile, although it is often contaminated by normal urethral organisms during micturition.

Inflammation

Inflammation is due to infection which, in this country, is invariably bacterial. Organisms usually enter the bladder along the urethra, and may extend up the ureters to produce pyelonephritis (above); they are usually derived from faecal contamination, and the most frequent is *Escherichia coli*. Cystitis, both acute and chronic, is much commoner in females, probably because their urethras are considerably shorter and wider.

Predisposing factors include obstruction with urinary stasis, paralysis, calculi, tumours and catheterisation.

Acute cystitis is usually limited to mucosa and submucosa. There may be ulceration and an overlying acute inflammatory exudate; local haemorrhage may present as haematuria. An intense polymorph infiltrate is seen, and polymorphs, together with causative organisms, are present in the urine. Resolution usually occurs, particularly with appropriate antibiotic therapy and removal of any predisposing factors, but recurrence rates are high.

Chronic cystitis may follow acute cystitis, especially if predisposing factors persist, or arise de novo. There is variable transmural chronic inflammation and fibrosis; in severe, long standing cases the bladder is thickened, inelastic and contracted, with a considerably reduced capacity. Rarely, it is due to tuberculosis; this represents intraluminal spread, usually from renal infection. In some areas, particularly the Middle East, schistosomiasis (also known as bilharziasis—infestation by *Schistosoma haematobium*) is a common cause.

Tumours

Malignant bladder tumours account for almost 4% of all malignancies, and over 90% are from transitional epithelium.

Transitional cell tumours arise anywhere in the urinary tract lined by transitional epithelium— they are mainly in the bladder, but may also develop in renal pelvis, ureters and proximal urethra. Most present between 50 and 70 years of age, and are about three times commoner in men. Unlike epithelial tumours elsewhere, the distinction here between benign and malignant neoplasms is blurred and difficult to define; indeed, some authorities do not accept a separate entity of benign transitional cell papilloma, and those who do acknowledge that it is very rare. This is because all transitional cell tumours possess a very great tendency for local recurrence and because affected patients have a very high risk of developing further such tumours elsewhere in their bladder or urinary tract; these two features reflect the so-called 'unstable urothelium'.

Aetiology. The male predominance reflects an

association with industrial chemical exposure, particularly aniline dye and rubber workers; specific carcinogens include the naphthylamines and benzidine. Cigarette smokers show an increased incidence, and schistosomiasis also predisposes.

Lesions. Transitional tumours are usually papillary, with frond-like processes projecting into the lumen, but many, particularly when less well differentiated, also have much more solid areas. Histologically, a spectrum of differentiation may be seen, from the rare papilloma with a thin covering of regular transitional cells to a solid, pleomorphic and hyperchromatic poorly differentiated tumour with frequent mitoses. Often, the urinary tract epithelium elsewhere shows chronic inflammation, and may be dysplastic.

Clinical. Most patients have haematuria which is usually painless and present throughout micturition. Many develop symptoms from associated infection, some show obstruction of ureters (to produce hydroureter and hydronephrosis) or of urethra (to cause urinary retention). Cytological urine screening may detect asymptomatic cases either as microscopic haematuria or from exfoliated tumour cells.

Spread. This may be direct into muscle and adjacent structures, or lymphatic to regional iliac and para-aortic lymph nodes. Haematogenous dissemination occurs, but is usually late.

Prognosis. This is influenced considerably by both histological differentiation and extent of spread at presentation (i.e. grade and stage). With superficial, well-differentiated tumours, 5-year survival is about 80%; with widespread, undifferentiated neoplasms, it is less than 30%.

URETHRA

Normal

The male urethra is 18–20 cm in length, and extends from bladder to distal penis. It is lined almost entirely by transitional epithelium, and conveys urine and semen to the outside world. In contrast, the female urethra is much shorter (about 4 cm long) and lined mostly by squamous epithelium.

Inflammation

Two types are described below, but some inevitably accompanies all ascending urinary tract infections, and is therefore always associated with cystitis.

Gonorrhoea, infection by *Neisseria gonorrhoeae* (gonococcus), is common and its incidence is increasing. It is acquired during sexual intercourse—that is, it is a venereal disease. Organisms initially colonise the anterior urethra to produce acute inflammation and a purulent exudate; without adequate antibiotic treatment they may spread to the posterior urethra (to produce a more chronic inflammatory response with fibrosis), other genital organs (e.g. prostate, epididymis, Fallopian tubes and ovaries) or elsewhere via the blood stream (e.g. joints and tendon sheaths).

Non-bacterial (non-specific) urethritis implies non-gonococcal inflammation. It is usually venereal, and many are thought to be due to *Chlamydia*. There is variable acute inflammation and haematogenous dissemination may produce conjunctivitis and arthritis (*Reiter's syndrome*).

Obstruction

Obstruction may be due to congenital, postinflammatory (usually gonococcal) or post-traumatic fibrous strictures: in males, prostatic hyperplasia and prostatic carcinoma (below) are common causes. It produces urine retention with, in more severe cases, bladder dilatation, hydroureters and bilateral hydronephrosis, and predisposes to ascending infections.

Prostatic hyperplasia, to some degree, is almost inevitable after middle age; it affects both glands and intervening fibromuscular stroma, and produces nodular enlargement. Aetiology is unknown, but androgen:oestrogen imbalance is probably a factor. Often, it is asymptomatic; symptoms, when present, usually relate to difficulties with micturition and urinary obstruction.

Prostatic carcinoma is fairly common, particularly in older men, and is an adenocarcinoma. Although it often co-exists with hyperplasia, this association is probably fortuitous, and its aetiology remains unknown. It has an unusual tendency to produce bone metastases, particularly in the lumbar spine, which usually stimulate local new bone formation—that is, they are osteosclerotic (Chapter 22).

DENTAL ASPECTS

Patients in chronic renal failure may show various oral changes, including erythema, ulceration and oral keratosis (Chapter 15). These abnormalities gradually disappear following correction of uraemia by regular dialysis.

Reference has already been made in Chapter 17 to the increased susceptibility of renal dialysis patients to hepatitis B virus infection.

Reiter's syndrome is often associated with oral abnormalities, for example, erythematous patches which may be surrounded by whitish serpiginous borders.

19

Endocrine diseases

Pituitary
Normal
Anterior pituitary
Posterior pituitary
Thyroid
Normal
Non-toxic goitre

Hypofunction
Hyperfunction
Tumours
Parathyroids
Normal
Hypofunction
Hyperfunction

Tumours
Adrenals
Normal
Cortical hypofunction
Cortical hyperfunction
Adrenal medulla

INTRODUCTION

Endocrine glands are important regulators of normal physiology. Each manufactures one or more hormones, and secretes them directly into the blood stream to affect distant organs or tissues.

Complex interrelationships exist between different glands and different hormones, and between endocrine and nervous systems via the hypothalamic/pituitary axis.

PITUITARY

Normal

The pituitary gland, in conjunction with the hypothalamus of the brain, plays a major role in controlling the endocrine system. Anatomically, it consists of two parts, *anterior* (adenohypophysis) and *posterior* (neurohypophysis). The *hypothalamus* acts as a regulator of both anterior and posterior pituitary secretory activity by producing peptides which stimulate or inhibit hormone secretion.

Anterior pituitary

The anterior pituitary is composed of two major cell groups according to staining affinity—*chromophils* and *chromophobes*.

Chromophils are traditionally divided into acidophils and basophils, but with more recent immunohistological techniques it is possible to identify individual cells containing specific hormones: adrenocorticotrophic hormone (ACTH); thyroid-stimulating hormone (TSH); melanocyte-stimulating hormone (MSH); growth hormone (GH); follicle-stimulating hormone (FSH); luteinising hormone in the female (LH); interstitial-cell-stimulating hormone in the male (ICSH); prolactin.

Hypofunction

Pituitary dwarfism (Lorain–Levi syndrome) results from reduced growth hormone production in childhood; other hormones may also be deficient. In one-third of cases a pituitary or brain tumour is present, but in the others no cause can be found. Impaired growth is usually noticed at an early age, and tooth development and eruption are delayed; in the absence of gonadotrophins, puberty does not occur.

Frolich's syndrome is stunting of growth, obesity with feminine distribution of fat, arrested sexual development and mental retardation due to abnormalities of the hypothalamus and/or anterior pituitary; possible causes include brain tumours and chromophobe adenomas.

Simmond's disease describes adult hypopituitarism, and includes ischaemic necrosis following postpartum haemorrhage (*Sheehan's syndrome*). Clinical features are variable and reflect consequent hypofunction of other endocrine organs.

Hyperfunction

Hyperfunction usually indicates an actively secreting pituitary adenoma.

Gigantism arises in children before bone epiphyses have fused. Excessive growth hormone secretion induces marked skeletal growth, and there is also a corresponding increase in size of internal organs (e.g. heart and liver).

Acromegaly occurs in adults after epiphyses have fused. Excess growth hormone leads to an increase in thickness of soft tissues and periosteal ossification which produces thickened bones. Overgrowth of the mandible (prognathism) is marked; malar bones and supra-orbital ridges are prominent and hands and feet are enlarged.

Cushing's syndrome of pituitary origin can be due to an adenoma or hyperplasia of basophil cells producing excess ACTH (see below).

Posterior pituitary

Posterior pituitary is associated with two hormones, vasopressin and oxytocin, both of which are synthesised in the hypothalamus, and modified and stored in the posterior pituitary.

Vasopressin (antidiuretic hormone, ADH) controls renal tubule permeability and hence urine concentration. ADH deficiency, normally caused by hypothalamic damage from head injury, glioma, metastatic tumours or encephalitis (Chapter 24), produces diabetes insipidus and is characterised by a large volume of dilute urine (polyuria) and excessive thirst (polydypsia).

Oxytocin causes uterine smooth muscle contraction and breast milk expulsion during lactation. It is widely used to induce labour.

THYROID

Normal

The thyroid is a bilobed gland with a central isthmus, and weighs approximately 25 g. It consists of follicles lined by cuboidal epithelium responsible for producing the iodine-containing hormones *tri-iodothyronine* (T_3) and *thyroxine* (T_4) and filled with thyroglobulin as colloid. Thyroid hormones influence intracellular transmembrane transport and enzyme activity, and thus stimulate cell metabolism. Another secretory cell (C cell) is present, either singly amongst follicular cells or as small aggregates in interfollicular spaces; it produces *calcitonin*, which lowers plasma calcium levels and promotes urinary phosphate excretion.

Non-toxic goitre

Non-toxic (simple) goitre is thyroid enlargement *not* associated with increased thyroid hormone secretion (hence 'non-toxic'). Dietary iodine deficiency is probably the chief aetiological factor; this impairs thyroid hormone synthesis and secretion, thus increasing pituitary TSH production. Prolonged TSH stimulation causes thyroid enlargement by producing nodules of large colloid-distended follicles with varying degrees of necrosis, haemorrhage and calcification—a *nodular colloid goitre*. In severe iodine lack, the hyperplastic changes are marked, producing a *diffuse* or *parenchymatous goitre*.

Hypofunction (hypothyroidism)

In children, it causes *cretinism*. The child may appear normal at birth but within weeks develops abnormalities including a protruding tongue and abdomen, mental deficiency and delayed dental development.

In adults, it produces *myxoedema*, with a reduced basal metabolic rate, lethargy, apathy and progressive non-pitting oedema due to increased subcutaneous tissue mucoproteins; thus, the tongue enlarges and the skin becomes 'puffy'. Histologically, the gland consists of fibrous tissue in which occasional atrophic acini are embedded.

Hashimoto's disease is an *autoimmune thyroiditis*; thyroid-specific antibodies are found in the serum of affected patients, and about half are hypothyroid. The gland shows a dense lymphoid cell infiltrate with fibrosis and loss of thyroid tissue.

Hyperfunction (hyperthyroidism, thyrotoxicosis)

In *Graves' disease* (exophthalmic goitre), diffuse enlargement is caused by a circulating inappropriate thyroid stimulator (an autoantibody) which reacts with and activates cell surface receptors for TSH. There is a rise in metabolic rate, increased heart rate, palpitations, nervousness and weight loss despite an excessive appetite. Exophthalmos (prominence of eyes) is common, and reflects fatty infiltration of retro-orbital tissues.

Toxic adenoma is uncommon. The hyperthyroidism produced is usually mild, and does not cause exophthalmos.

Toxic nodular goitre occurs occasionally in patients with a long-standing non-toxic goitre; again, the hyperthyroidism is mild.

Tumours

Adenomas are common, and may be multiple. They usually present a follicular pattern histologically, and sometimes they may be difficult to distinguish from nodules of a nodular colloid goitre.

Adenocarcinomas, derived from thyroid epithelium, are uncommon. Two forms, reflecting basic structural features, are recognised (*papillary* and *follicular*).

Medullary carcinoma is rare. It is derived from C cells, which are part of the APUD system (Chapter 10).

PARATHYROIDS

Normal

The parathyroids are four small glands usually lying behind the thyroid. They consist of chief, water-clear (secretory variants of chief) and oxyphil cells. They produce parathyroid hormone (PTH) which maintains normal ionised calcium levels in body fluids by acting at three sites—bone (stimulating osteoclastic resorption), renal tubules (increasing calcium ion reabsorption) and small intestine (by increasing calcium absorption).

Hypofunction

Inadequate PTH production occurs under three circumstances: *accidental surgical removal* of one or more parathyroids during thyroidectomy, *idiopathic (familial) hypoparathyroidism* resulting from gradual autoimmune destruction and *congenital deficiency* due to parathyroid hypoplasia. There is a decrease in plasma ionised calcium, which increases nerve excitability and, if severe, causes spasm and twitching of muscles (*tetany*). Dentition abnormalities are common in children, including hypoplastic enamel and delayed eruption of teeth.

Hyperfunction

Primary hyperparathyroidism is due to diffuse hyperplasia, adenoma or carcinoma of chief cells.

There is increased PTH production resulting in raised plasma calcium levels (*hypercalcaemia*); excess calcium excreted in the urine causes *renal calculi*. Prolonged intense osteoclastic bone resorption produces destructive cystic lesions (*osteitis fibrosa cystica*) often accompanied by bone pain and an increased tendency to pathological fractures; sometimes, a tumour-like mass of osteoclasts and haemosiderin from focal haemorrhage ('*brown tumour*') develops, particularly in skull, jaw, ribs and spine. *Metastatic calcification* due to the hypercalcaemia can occur in kidneys, lungs and stomach (Chapter 7). Dental radiographs may show loss of lamina dura around teeth; although non-specific, this may be the first indication of hyperparathyroidism.

Secondary hyperparathyroidism is a compensatory increase in PTH secretion in response to low plasma calcium levels. It is most commonly associated with chronic renal failure, but may also complicate vitamin D deficiency and malabsorption syndrome.

Tertiary hyperparathyroidism is rare. It results from an autonomous adenoma developing in long-standing secondary hyperparathyroidism; PTH levels are greater than required, and plasma calcium becomes elevated.

Tumours

Adenomas are uncommon, *carcinoma* is very rare; both may cause hyperparathyroidism.

ADRENALS

Normal

Adrenals consist of two parts—*cortex* and *medulla*. The cortex has three zones—zona glomerulosa (producing aldosterone), zona fasciculata (corticosteroids) and zona reticularis (steroid sex hormones); the medulla produces adrenaline and noradrenaline.

Cortical hypofunction

Acute insufficiency occurs in individuals unable to increase corticosteroid production when exposed to sudden stress (e.g. severe trauma, haemorrhage or infection). This may be seen in patients on long term oral *steroid therapy* when such treatment is stopped abruptly, as these circulating steroids depress pituitary ACTH secretion and thus produce adrenal atrophy; it is usual, therefore, to reduce steroid dosage gradually over a long period or to administer ACTH before withdrawing steroid therapy.

Chronic insufficiency occurs in *Addison's disease* (when the glands are destroyed by an autoimmune process) and with bilateral replacement by tuberculosis, secondary tumour deposits or amyloidosis. Affected patients show low blood pressure, loss of appetite and weight, low plasma sodium (hyponatraemia) and high plasma potassium (hyperkalaemia). An unusual feature is the increase in melanin pigmentation of skin and oral mucosa, possibly due to excess pituitary MSH and ACTH production.

Cortical hyperfunction

Cushing's syndrome is caused by excessive production (or administration) of glucocorticoids, and characterised by moon-shaped face, obesity, hyperglycaemia, osteoporosis, hypertension and muscle wasting. It may be due to a basophil adenoma of the anterior pituitary producing excess ACTH, hyperplasia or an adenoma of the adrenal cortex itself or ectopic ACTH production by tumours (e.g. oat cell carcinoma of lung or thymoma).

Conn's syndrome (*primary aldosteronism*) results from hyperplasia or an adenoma of the zona glomerulosa. The excess aldosterone produces abnormal sodium retention (causing hypertension) and potassium loss.

Virilism in females and the *adrenogenital syndrome* (precocious puberty) in children can occur with an adrenal adenoma producing excess male sex hormones (androgens).

Adrenal medulla

The adrenal medulla is derived from neural crest cells which differentiate into chromaffin and autonomic ganglion cells, and it secretes the catecholamine hormones adrenaline and noradrenaline. The main lesions are the tumours arising from its various cell types.

Phaeochromocytoma occurs mostly as a solitary neoplasm and is an APUD cell tumour (APUDoma—Chapter 10). It comprises polyhedral cells, many of which give the chromaffin reaction (staining brownish-yellow when fixed in dichromate). It produces, usually intermittently at first, excess catecholamines, which cause paroxysmal hypertension, nervousness, tremors, palpitations and headache. Familial bilateral phaeochromocytomas associated with medullary carcinoma of thyroid are sometimes categorised as *multiple endocrine neoplasia syndrome*; there may also be multiple neuromas of the oral mucosa.

Neuroblastoma and its differentiated counterpart *ganglioneuroma* are derived from nerve cells and are tumours of childhood; both may secrete catecholamines.

20

Haematological diseases

Normal
Red blood cells
Dyshaemopoietic anaemias
Haemolytic anaemias

White blood cells
Leucocytosis and leucopaenia
Myeloproliferative disorders
Bone marrow neoplasms
Plasma cell neoplasms

Leukaemia
Haemorrhagic diseases
Normal haemostasis
Haemorrhagic states
Dental aspects

Normal

Haemopoiesis (formation of blood cells) in the normal adult takes place in red bone marrow; in the fetus and in some disease states it is also extramedullary (e.g. in liver and spleen). Red cells, white cells and platelets share a common ancestor, the pluripotent haemopoietic stem cell, which gives rise to daughter cells that increase in number by undergoing amplification division until they become restricted in differentiation potential to a single cell line. Control of these progenitor populations is complex, but an important factor influencing red cell production is erythropoietin released by the kidney in response to hypoxia. Some normal values are shown in Table 20.1; as figures vary slightly between laboratories, students should always use those provided by their local hospital. Definitions of parameters used include:

Haematocrit or *packed cell volume* (PCV) is the proportion of red cells in a given volume of blood.

Mean corpuscular volume (MCV)

$$= \frac{\text{haematocrit}}{\text{number of red cells/litre}} \quad \text{fl}$$

Mean corpuscular haemoglobin (MCH)

$$= \frac{\text{haemoglobin (g/dl)}}{\text{number of red cells/dl}} \quad \text{pg}$$

Mean corpuscular haemoglobin concentration (MCHC)

$$= \frac{\text{haemoglobin (g/dl)}}{\text{haematocrit}} \quad \text{g/dl}$$

RED BLOOD CELLS (ERYTHROCYTES)

Anaemia is a reduction in haemoglobin concentration in the blood. It is usually accompanied by a fall in the red cell count, and represents an imbalance between red cell production and destruction. All anaemias share the same non-specific *signs and symptoms*, including lethargy, giddiness, breathlessness, pallor of skin, mucosae and conjunctivae and increase in heart rate and force. There may be erythropoietin-induced enhanced haemopoiesis (i.e. bone marrow hyperplasia) as a compensating mechanism, although this may be unsuccessful. Anaemic patients do not show central cyanosis as their haemoglobin, although decreased in amount, is usually well

Table 20.1 Normal blood cell values

Haemoglobin
    Adult males   13.0–18.0 g/dl
    Adult females 11.5–16.5 g/dl

Red blood cells
    Adult males $4.5–6.5 \times 10^{12}/l$
    Adult females $3.8–5.8 \times 10^{12}/l$

Red cell values
    Haematocrit (packed cell volume, PCV):
        Adult males   0.40–0.54
        Adult females   0.37–0.47
    Mean corpuscular volume (MCV) 80–97 fl
    Mean corpuscular haemoglobin (MCH) 27–32 pg
    Mean corpuscular haemoglobin concentration (MCHC) 31–35 g/dl

White blood cells
    Total number $4–11 \times 10^9/l$

Differential white blood cell count
    Neutrophils $2.0–7.5 \times 10^9/l$ (40–75% of total number)
    Lymphocytes $1.5–4.0 \times 10^9/l$ (20–45% of total number)
    Monocytes $0.2–0.8 \times 10^9/l$ (2–10% of total number)
    Eosinophils $0.04–0.4 \times 10^9/l$ (1–6% of total number)
    Basophils $<0.1 \times 10^9/l$ (< 1% of total number)

Platelets
    Total number $150–400 \times 10^9/l$

oxygenated. Long-standing cases may show fatty change (Chapter 2) of liver and heart. A classification is shown in Table 20.2; they can also be considered according to cell haemoglobin content (normochromic = normal, hypochromic = reduced: note that hyperchromia does not exist) and size (normocytic = normal, microcytic = reduced, macrocytic = increased).

Table 20.2 Classification of anaemias

Decreased production of red cells
  Dyshaemopoietic anaemias
    Iron deficiency anaemia
    Megaloblastic anaemia
  Hypoplastic and aplastic anaemias

Increased destruction of red cells
  Haemolytic—defective red cells
              Hereditary spherocytosis
              Enzyme abnormalities
              Haemoglobinopathies
                Sickle cell disease
                Thalassaemia
         —abnormality extrinsic to red cells:
              Antibodies to red cells:
                Haemolytic disease of the newborn
                Incompatible blood transfusion
                Autoimmune disease
              Miscellaneous

Dyshaemopoietic anaemias

Dyshaemopoietic anaemias are caused by a deficiency of one or more substances necessary for normal red cell production—iron, folic acid and vitamin B_{12}. Normal levels are shown in Table 20.3.

Iron deficiency anaemia. This is the commonest, and is the result of a negative iron balance, that is, a greater loss than can be compensated for by increased intestinal absorption. The commonest cause is *chronic blood loss*, as with repeated gastrointestinal tract haemorrhages (e.g. peptic ulcer, aspirin ingestion, carcinoma and hookworm infestation in tropical areas) and during menstruation (women have lower iron stores than men and this physiological loss is a frequent cause of anaemia). Other causes are *increased demand* (e.g. during childhood and pregnancy), *malabsorption* from the gastrointestinal tract (Chapter 16), *inadequate dietary intake* and *disturbances of iron metabolism*. As iron balance deteriorates, stores are mobilised in an attempt to keep the serum iron (and hence iron available for haemopoiesis)

Table 20.3 Normal biochemical values of substances necessary for red blood cell production

Serum Iron	7–29 μmol/l
Total iron-binding capacity (TIBC)	45–70 μmol/l
% Saturation $\dfrac{\text{serum iron}}{\text{TIBC}}$ =	33% approximately
Folate—red cell	200–600 μg/l
serum	3–16 μg/l
Serum B_{12}	150–900 ng/l

normal. Once the stores are depleted, serum iron falls and TIBC rises; hence saturation falls markedly, and a value less than 16% indicates iron deficiency. During early iron deficiency, sufficient iron reaches the marrow for normal haemopoiesis, and so haemoglobin and red cell counts are normal. If untreated, there is progression to anaemia, with a fall in haemoglobin, red cell number, MCH and MCHC; a blood film shows the small, poorly staining red cells of this microcytic, hypochromic anaemia. White cell and platelet counts remain normal; the marrow is hyperplastic. Clinically, in addition to general signs and symptoms of anaemia described earlier, there may be specific features, including *koilonychia* (spoon-shaped finger nails), a reduction in prominence of filiform papillae on the tongue, *angular cheilitis, recurrent oral ulceration* (Chapter 15) and Paterson–Kelly syndrome (Chapter 16).

Megaloblastic anaemia. This is characterised by megaloblasts in marrow and macrocytes in peripheral blood; it is caused by lack of folic acid or vitamin B_{12}. Causes of folic acid deficiency include *dietary insufficiency* (e.g. in the elderly, alcoholics and infants), *malabsorption* (coeliac disease being the most important example), *drugs* interfering with folic acid metabolism (e.g. methotrexate in cancer treatment and phenytoin) and *increased body demand* (e.g. increased cell production states such as pregnancy and neoplasia). Causes of vitamin B_{12} deficiency include *malabsorption*, *'blind loop' syndrome* (where B_{12} is absorbed by excess jejunal bacteria following intestinal stasis), infestation by the *tapeworm Diphyllobothrium latum, dietary deficiency* and *lack of intrinsic factor* (IF), the gastric cofactor required for B_{12} absorption (seen after total gastrectomy and in autoimmune gastritis; the latter produces the commonest and best-known example—*pernicious anaemia*—where circulating antibodies to parietal cells (the source of IF) are present in 90% of cases and antibodies to IF are present in gastric secretions in 50%). In megaloblastic anaemias, the peripheral blood shows enlarged red cells (macrocytes), variations in red cell size (anisocytosis) and shape (poikilocytosis), and some reduction in white cells and platelets. The MCV is increased but the MCHC is normal (because MCHC rises in proportion to MCV); haemoglobin and red cell counts are lowered, the latter often markedly. Differences between megaloblastic and iron deficiency anaemias are shown in Table 20.4. The marrow is hyperplastic and megaloblastic—that is, all cells show an imbalance between nuclear and cytoplasmic maturation, with accumulation of large immature cells including nucleated red cells (megaloblasts). Similar abnormalities of platelet and leucocyte precursors also exist. Clinically, untreated cases show loss of lingual filiform and fungiform papillae which, together with generalised mucosal epithelial atrophy, produces the classical red, raw, 'beefy' tongue rarely seen nowadays.

Neurological abnormalities associated with B_{12} but not folate deficiency include subacute combined degeneration of the spinal cord and a peripheral neuropathy (Chapter 24).

Hypoplastic and aplastic anaemia. A significant reduction in haemopoietic marrow (hypoplasia, or, if severe, 'aplasia') results in a decrease in red cells, white cells and platelets—that is, a pancytopaenia, with normochromic, normocytic anaemia, agranulocytosis and thrombocytopaenia. Causes include marrow destruction by *irradiation* or *cytotoxic drugs* (the latter represents a side effect of cancer treatment but may also be an idiosyncratic reaction to other chemotherapeutic agents e.g. chloramphenicol, sulphonamides and antirheumatic drugs) and

marrow replacement by *myelofibrosis* or *tumour infiltration* (usually leukaemias); about 50% of cases are *idiopathic*.

Haemolytic anaemias

In this group, red cells have a reduced lifespan due either to an intracellular defect making them more fragile, or to extracellular haemolytic factors enhancing their destruction in the reticulo-endothelial system, mainly the spleen, and occasionally the circulation (see Table 20.2). The marrow responds by becoming hyperplastic, and reticulocytes (immature red cells) enter the circulation, sometimes in large numbers. Normochromic, normocytic anaemia is usual. Increased haemoglobin catabolism causes a rise in plasma bilirubin and, if severe, acholuric jaundice (Chapter 17). Intravascular red cell destruction can lead to haemoglobinaemia and even haemoglobinuria.

Haemolysis due to defective red cells

Hereditary spherocytosis. This is a common, inherited (autosomal dominant) abnormality of red cell membrane metabolism, producing cells that are spherical and thus more easily trapped and broken down in splenic sinusoids. There is usually a mild anaemia but episodes of severe anaemia, fever and jaundice occur. Splenectomy is beneficial (the spleen is markedly enlarged at operation) but the basic defect remains. Susceptibility of the cells to destruction is shown by their increased osmotic fragility in saline.

Enzyme defects. Glucose-6-phosphate dehydrogenase (G6PD) deficiency is an inherited sex-linked condition which is very common in Negro and Mediterranean peoples. It allows haemoglobin to be oxidised and denatured easily, and may happen after eating the *Vicia fava* bean (which contains oxidants) or following phenacetin or antimalarial drug treatment.

Haemoglobinopathies. Haemoglobin comprises haem and globin, the latter containing two pairs of polypeptide chains. In normal adults, HbA (two α, two β chains) and a small amount of HbA_2 (two α, two δ chains) are present. Several abnormal haemoglobins affecting either α or β chains exist and collectively are known as haemoglobinopathies.

Table 20.4 Summary of differences between iron deficiency and megaloblastic anaemias

	Iron deficiency	Megaloblastic
Haemoglobin	Much reduced	Reduced
Red cell count	Reduced	Much reduced
Abnormal red cell shape	Absent	Present
MCV	Reduced	Increased
MCHC	Reduced	Normal
White cells and platelets	Normal	Reduced

Sickle cell disease presents as homozygous, sickle cell anaemia (affecting less than 1% of American Negroes) or heterozygous, sickle cell trait (up to 20%). The abnormal haemoglobin (HbS) which follows substitution of glutamine by valine at position 6 in β chains, accounts for 75–100% of haemoglobin in homozygotes and up to 45% in heterozygotes. When deoxygenated, it distorts the red cells into sickle-like forms which are trapped and broken down in the enlarged spleen. These can form aggregates and block small blood vessels to produce infarcts anywhere in the body. Sickling occurs spontaneously in homozygotes but only when oxygen levels are reduced (as in general anaesthesia or at high altitudes) in heterozygotes. Clinically, the homozygous form is usually seen in childhood; haemolytic anaemia, pain from infarcts in bone etc., fever and recurrent infections are common, and patients tend to die in early adult life. On the other hand, heterozygotes can be symptomless, and so, because of its high incidence, all Negroes who require a general anaesthetic should be investigated routinely for its presence. For some unknown reason, HbS confers some resistance to malaria.

Thalassaemia is a group of diseases with inadequate synthesis of α or β globin chains. In *α thalassaemia*, reduced α chain synthesis leads to a decrease in HbA and HbA$_2$ with the compensatory appearance of Hb Barts (four γ chains) and HbH (four β chains). *Beta thalassaemia* shows a decrease in HbA, with an increase in HbA$_2$ and HbF (fetal haemoglobin—two α, two γ chains), both of which lack β chains and are therefore unaffected. No abnormal haemoglobins are produced. In both types, red cells have a reduced survival, but, unlike hereditary spherocytosis, their osmotic fragility is reduced. Homozygous and heterozygous forms exist; the former (thalassaemia major) causes severe anaemia, splenomegaly and haemosiderosis, with death at an early age: the latter (thalassaemia minor) may be asymptomatic or produce a mild but resistant microcytic hypochromic anaemia.

Haemolysis due to extrinsic factors

Haemolytic disease of the newborn (HDN). This occurs when a rhesus negative (Rh−) woman produces antibodies to Rh+ fetal red cells, which may enter her circulation during childbirth. Although the firstborn child is unaffected, IgG antibodies cross the placenta during subsequent pregnancies to destroy Rh+ fetal red cells and to produce HDN. This will occur in every subsequent pregnancy if the father is homozygous Rh+. HDN in its mildest form produces fetal anaemia and transient jaundice—*congenital haemolytic anaemia*; if severe, the elevated unconjugated bilirubin levels may cause permanent brain damage (*kernicterus*) and even death in utero from severe anaemia and cardiac failure (*hydrops fetalis*). Treatment includes antenatal or postnatal exchange transfusion of the affected infant and prophylactic administration to the mother of rhesus antibodies shortly after delivery to prevent her developing her own antibodies.

Others. Other extrinsic causes include *autoimmune* (with cytotoxic autoantibodies produced against red cells; this may be primary or complicate drug treatment, collagen diseases and syphilis), *malaria* (in which the parasite invades and lyses red cells), *bacterial toxaemia* (e.g. *Clostridium welchii*), *chronic lead poisoning* and *mechanical damage* within the circulation of the feet during long marches or following entrapment in fibrin deposits within small vessels damaged in various conditions such as malignant hypertension.

WHITE BLOOD CELLS (LEUCOCYTES)

Leucocytes comprise three types of polymorphs (neutrophil, eosinophil and basophil), monocytes and lymphocytes. As any increase (*leucocytosis*) or decrease (*leucopaenia*) in circulating white cells is invariably associated with a change in the proportions of the different types, it is important that absolute rather than relative values are obtained and considered (see Table 20.1).

Leucocytosis and leucopaenia

Neutrophil leucocytosis is usually due to bacterial infections; other causes include tissue necrosis (e.g. infarction), burns, crush injuries, corticosteroid excess and chronic myeloid leukaemia. *Neutrophil leucopaenia* (*neutropaenia*) can be due to marrow defects (replacement by leukaemia, fibrosis or metastatic tumour; idiosyncratic reactions to drugs; radiation), hypersplenism (enhanced breakdown by the spleen) or anaphylaxis. The term *agranulocytosis* applies when the neutropaenia is particularly severe. In *cyclical neutropaenia*, there is a cyclical fall in circulating neutrophils, and recurrent oral ulceration may follow (Chapter 15). Effects include infection by pathogenic and commensal organisms.

Eosinophil leucocytosis (*eosinophilia*) occurs in hypersensitivity states (e.g. asthma, hay fever, drug- and food-related allergies), parasitic infestations, some chronic skin diseases (e.g. dermatitis herpetiformis) and with certain neoplasms (e.g. Hodgkin's disease). *Eosinophil leucopaenia* can be drug induced (e.g. glucocorticosteroids) or due to marrow dysfunction (see neutrophil leucopaenia).

Monocytosis may be found in subacute infective endocarditis, infections (e.g. malaria, rickettsia-induced) and monocytic leukaemia.

Lymphocytosis occurs in infections (e.g. infectious mononucleosis, smallpox, syphilis and influenza) and chronic lymphocytic leukaemia. *Lymphopaenia* may follow cytotoxic or radiation treatment and occurs in immunodeficiency states.

Myeloproliferative disorders

Myeloproliferative disorders are characterised by uncontrolled, non-physiological proliferation of bone marrow constituents, and include *polycythaemia vera* in which the erythroid cell line is particularly affected, *myeloid leukaemia* from uncontrolled proliferation of granulocytes, *thrombocythaemia* with increased platelet production and *myelofibrosis* in which the marrow becomes replaced by fibrous tissue. These conditions can occur independently of each other, but they may overlap, with transition from one to another.

Polycythaemia

Polycythaemia is an absolute increase in the red cell count.

In *polycythaemia vera* (*primary polycythaemia*), it can be $7-9 \times 10^{12}/l$, with a greatly increased haematocrit (60–70%) and haemoglobin; in fact, the latter may be so high that central cyanosis is common. White cell and platelet numbers are usually also raised. Patients are middle aged or elderly, with dusky, florid features, hypertension, and a bleeding or thrombotic tendency, the last producing multiple organ infarcts; some develop gout due to increased turnover of uric acid from nuclear protein metabolism.

In *secondary polycythaemia*, red cells are increased by erythropoietin-induced stimulation of erythrocytosis, causes of which include chronic hypoxia (e.g. high altitudes, respiratory diseases, congenital heart diseases) and renal or extrarenal production by neoplasms; white cells and platelets are normal.

Myelofibrosis

Myelofibrosis is a disease of the elderly in which fibrous tissue replacement of haemopoietic marrow produces anaemia. Extramedullary haemopoiesis in spleen and liver leads to an increase in their size. Immature white and red cells appear in the circulation, hence the so-called *leucoerythroblastic* appearance in blood films. Ultimately, a pancytopaenia develops.

Myeloid leukaemia and *thrombocythaemia* are considered below.

BONE MARROW NEOPLASMS

These are primary or secondary. Metastatic deposits are common, and often originate from bronchus, breast, thyroid or malignant melanoma. Primary neoplasms include those of *plasma cells* and the *leukaemias*.

Plasma cell neoplasms

Multiple myeloma affects mainly the middle aged and elderly; M:F ratio is approximately 2:1. Neoplastic plasma cells are present in many sites in different bones, with skull lesions in 70% and jaw involvement in 30%. Radiographically, these areas are seen as well-delineated, 'punched-out' defects. Skeletal lesions may cause vertebral body collapse, pathological fractures and hypercalcaemia; anaemia, infections and haemorrhage develop as normal haemopoietic marrow becomes replaced by neoplastic cells. As the disease is monoclonal, there is an increase in serum immunoglobulin levels of one class, usually IgG. There may also be excess light chain production; if so, it invariably appears in the urine as *Bence–Jones protein*, which can precipitate in renal tubules and lead eventually to renal failure. Amyloidosis, of primary type, is another complication of light chain production (Chapter 7). Rarely, a single focus of neoplastic plasma cells, indistinguishable from those in multiple myeloma, is seen as a *solitary plasmacytoma*; it usually affects bone, but may be seen in soft tissues. Affected patients will probably develop multiple myeloma eventually, although this may take 20 years or more. Because of their small size and limited distribution, solitary lesions are rarely associated with Bence–Jones proteinuria or hypergammaglobulinaemia. Histologically, it may be difficult to distinguish monoclonal, neoplastic plasma cell infiltrates from polyclonal, reactive ones, and so techniques to demonstrate the heavy and light chains present may be used on tissue sections; in reactive infiltrates both κ and λ light chains and several heavy chains are present, whereas neoplastic infiltrates show only κ or λ and a single heavy chain.

Waldenstrom's macroglobulinaemia affects elderly males, and is a low grade B cell neoplasm producing high circulating IgM levels. As the bone marrow is replaced by neoplastic cells, anaemia, infections and haemorrhage develop.

Leukaemia

Leukaemia is the neoplastic proliferation of leucocyte precursors in the bone marrow; typically, the cells appear in peripheral blood (hence the name) and eventually infiltrate other organs. It is classified as acute or chronic and according to cell types involved. Distinction from lymphomas is sometimes blurred (Chapter 21), and overlap may occur.

Causes include *genetic factors* (e.g. the abnormal 22 'Philadelphia' chromosome in 90% of patients with chronic myeloid leukaemia), *irradiation* (e.g. atomic bomb survivors), *chemicals* (e.g. benzene) and, possibly, *viruses*.

Acute leukaemia can occur at any age, with acute lymphoblastic mainly in children and acute myeloblastic in adults. It is rapidly progressive and fatal if untreated; chemotherapy produces a much better prognosis, especially in children. Presenting signs and symptoms are those of bone-marrow replacement—anaemia, bleeding and infection; many, therefore, have oral manifestations, including gingival enlargement and bleeding, ulceration, mucosal petechiae and cervical lymphadenopathy. The peripheral blood usually shows an increase in white cells (often $20–50 \times 10^9/l$) with abnormal, immature forms; in approximately one-third of cases the white cell count is normal (aleukaemic leukaemia) although abnormal cells are present. The marrow is hypercellular, with numerous blast cells but fewer red cell and platelet precursors.

Chronic myeloid leukaemia usually affects older people. It develops slowly to produce anaemia and bleeding; often it ultimately transforms into acute myeloblastic leukaemia. The white cell count can be as high as $500 \times 10^9/l$, due mainly to excess mature and immature neutrophil polymorphs. In the hypercellular marrow, granulocyte precursors predominate.

Chronic lymphocytic leukaemia also affects older people. The marrow gradually becomes replaced by neoplastic lymphocytes, and the blood may contain $50–250 \times 10^9/l$ leucocytes, mostly lymphocytes. Clinically, in addition to anaemia, haemorrhage and infection, lymphadenopathy usually occurs early in the disease. Progression is often slow, and acute transformation does not occur.

HAEMORRHAGIC DISEASES

Normal haemostasis

Arrest of haemorrhage after vascular injury depends on blood vessel constriction, formation of a platelet mass at the damaged site and blood coagulation (fibrin deposition); this is then followed by clot retraction, activation of fibrinolytic mechanisms and, finally, fibroblastic and endothelial proliferation.

Platelets adhere to damaged endothelium and exposed collagen, and aggregate, under the influence of adenosine diphosphate (ADP), to form a sticky plug. The factors they release initiate blood coagulation and clot retraction.

Blood coagulation (clotting) is by the cascade mechanism (Fig. 20.1) resulting in fibrin production. The *extrinsic pathway* is activated by factors, including thromboplastin, released by damaged cells; the *intrinsic pathway* is activated by contact with abnormal surfaces, including collagen. The fibrin clot is at first poorly formed but becomes compact and polymeric under the influence of factor XIII.

Fibrinolysis is achieved by activation of plasminogen, which breaks down fibrin to its degradation products (Fig. 20.1).

Haemorrhagic states

Abnormalities of platelets (number or function), vessel walls, clotting or fibrinolysis will result in abnormal haemorrhage. The bleeding time is increased if platelets are defective or if the vessel fails to contract, whereas an increased clotting time follows failure of coagulation. Bleeding can

be classified according to size: *purpura* is bleeding from capillaries, producing tiny haemorrhagic spots in skin and mucosae (*petechiae*); in contrast, *haematomas (bruises)* are large accumulations of blood, with local tissue displacement and swelling, caused by bleeding from large vessels. The latter do not necessarily indicate underlying haemorrhagic disease. Causes of haemorrhagic states are shown in Table 20.5.

Platelet abnormalities

Thrombocytopaenic purpura requires a large fall in platelets to below $20–40 \times 10^9/l$. It may be primary (idiopathic—see below) or secondary to *marrow insufficiency* (e.g. in megaloblastic or aplastic anaemias, myelofibrosis or following irradiation), *drugs* (e.g. Sedormid®) or *excess breakdown* (e.g. in hypersplenism or disseminated intravascular coagulation, where platelets are trapped by fibrin in vessels). *Idiopathic thrombocytopaenic purpura* is an autoimmune disease of young people in which antibodies are produced

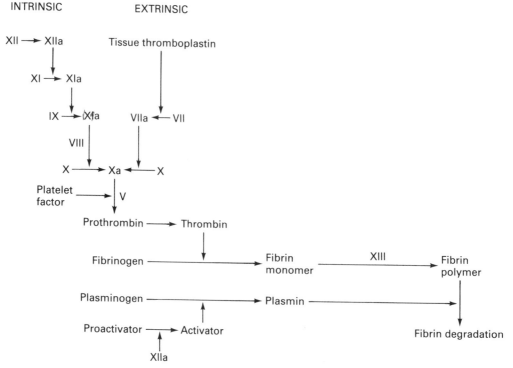

Fig. 20.1 Blood coagulation and fibrinolytic mechanisms (a = activated form; XIII = fibrin-stabilising factor; XII = Hageman factor; XI = plasma thromboplastin antecedent; X = Stuart Prower factor; IX = Christmas factor; VIII = antihaemophilic globulin; VII = Proconvertin; V = proaccelerin)

Table 20.5 Causes of haemorrhagic states

Platelets
   Thrombocytopaenia
   Thrombocythaemia
   Thrombocytopathia

Vessel wall
   Protein and vitamin C deficiency
   Local infection
   Henoch–Schönlein purpura
   Hereditary haemorrhagic telangiectasia

Coagulation factors
   Haemophilia
   Von Willebrand's disease
   Christmas disease
   Acquired defects

against platelets. Bleeding occurs into the skin and mouth, but severe intracerebral or gastro intestinal haemorrhages are also possible. It is usually self limiting, lasting a few months.

Thrombocythaemia is a myeloproliferative disorder characterised by increased platelet production. Although the platelet count is high, bleeding occurs because they are functionally defective.

Thrombocytopathia describes defective platelet function despite a normal platelet count. It may complicate uraemia or Waldenstrom's macroglobulinaemia.

Capillary wall abnormalities

Haemorrhage from capillary wall abnormalities is seen in protein and vitamin C deficiencies, and following local damage by infection and inflammation (e.g. meningococcal septicaemia and septic emboli, including subacute infective endocarditis).

Henoch–Schönlein purpura is a generalised hypersensitivity reaction which may follow streptococcal pharyngitis. Associated bleeding into skin and gastrointestinal tract, polyarthritis and glomerulonephritis are invariably transient.

Hereditary haemorrhagic telangiectasia is a rare, autosomal dominant abnormality of capillaries producing bleeding. Nose bleeds (epistaxes) are common, and repeated haemorrhage may cause iron deficiency anaemia.

Coagulation factor deficiencies

Haemophilia. This is a sex-linked, recessive deficiency of factor VIII. Females are carriers and half their sons are affected. Bleeding follows trivial injury, and joints are particularly affected by haemarthrosis leading to ankylosis and crippling deformities; haemorrhage into the floor of the mouth may cause breathing difficulties. Factor VIII levels should be increased to at least 30% of normal by giving purified factor VIII, fresh frozen plasma or cryoprecipitate containing factor VIII before surgical operations, including dental extractions, are attempted; antifibrinolytic agents (e.g. epsilon-aminocaproic acid) are also useful in contributing to haemostasis.

Von Willebrand's disease. This is an autosomal dominant condition of factor VIII deficiency combined with a capillary abnormality so that bleeding and clotting times are increased.

Christmas disease. This is a sex-linked, recessive deficiency of factor IX, and is similar clinically to haemophilia.

Others. Acquired defects usually involve several coagulation factors, many of which depend on vitamin K. The latter may be deficient in neonates (due to inadequate intestinal bacteria), malabsorption, liver failure and following treatment with anticoagulants of the coumarin group. Fibrinolytic mechanisms may be activated to such an extent that plasmin is produced within the circulation; usually this is due to disseminated intravascular coagulation produced by introduction of foreign material into the blood stream, severe infection, trauma or surgery. Intravascular clotting and/or haemorrhage result, with consequent shock.

DENTAL ASPECTS

Haematological diseases can affect appearance and function of oral mucosa in many ways. The dental surgeon must be familiar with them, as he will often be able to detect oral and facial abnormalities with an underlying haematological cause. Patients with recurrent oral infections or ulceration require investigations including a routine blood count. Signs and symptoms of anaemia together with its associated tongue changes, tendency for oral ulceration, impaired wound healing and general anaesthetic risk (especially sickle cell disease) should be recognised. Mouth involvement in leukaemia and haemorrhagic states, and jaw lesions in multiple myeloma are less common but important. Because of the risks of surgery and of developing antibodies to administered factor VIII, preventive dental care is an essential part of the management of haemophiliacs. It should be remembered that bleeding *from gingival margins* is almost always due to gingivitis and only rarely attributable to one of the haemorrhagic diseases listed in this chapter.

21

Diseases of the lymphoreticular system

Introduction
Lymph nodes
Normal
Lymphadenopathy
Neoplasms
Spleen

Normal
Splenomegaly
Neoplasms
Thymus
Normal
Neoplasms

INTRODUCTION

The lymphoreticular system comprises lymph nodes, spleen and thymus. It takes part in immune responses (Chapter 6) and, like liver and bone marrow, contains numerous macrophages, allowing an additional, non-immunological, phagocytic role.

LYMPH NODES

Normal

From afferent lymphatics, lymph enters peripheral sinuses between the outer capsule and cortex, and passes, via sinusoids, through the paracortex to the medulla, which it then leaves via efferent lymphatics. In the *cortex* are most of the B lymphocytes and numerous, discrete *lymphoid follicles*. Each follicle has a pale *germinal centre* (in which maturation of B cells occurs and where macrophages trap and process antigens) and a periphery or mantle of mature B lymphocytes. During B cell immunological reactions, the increase in number and size of lymphoid follicles produces cortical enlargement. The deeper *paracortex* contains most of the T lymphocytes and histiocytes; an increase in either produces enlargement of this zone. Postcapillary venules with prominent endothelial cells ('high endothelial venules') are found here, and they play an important role in lymphocyte traffic through the node. The *medulla*, through which lymph and lymphocytes drain, contains prominent sinusoids, which can appear dilated and prominent during reactive processes.

This structural complexity accounts for the wide variety of histological abnormalities in disease. Although some changes indicate specific diseases, frequently they are not pathognomonic of a single condition but are consistent with a wide range of aetiological factors, reflecting the central role which lymph nodes play in host defences.

Lymphadenopathy

Lymphadenopathy (lymph node enlargement) is usually inflammatory in origin—*acute and chronic lymphadenitis*—and this is invariably due to lymphatic drainage of the aetiological agent or its products to regional nodes. Clinically, the affected node is enlarged and painful, and in severe acute lymphadenitis it may be destroyed by suppuration, and pus may discharge on to overlying skin via a sinus track. Less commonly, lymphadenopathy is due to neoplasms—see below.

Infections

Bacterial infection may lead to suppuration and is usually due to staphylococci or streptococci.

Tuberculosis of cervical nodes was common before milk was pasteurised routinely; in primary infection, *Mycobacterium bovis* entered through the tonsil and drained to the deep cervical chain. Bronchial and hilar nodes are involved in pulmonary tuberculosis (primary complex), and mesenteric nodes in primary intestinal infection (Chapter 5). Results include caseation with discharge of necrotic material ('cold abscess' formation) and calcification.

In *cat-scratch disease*, unidentified micro-organisms enter the skin wound; the lymphadenitis with suppuration can be considerable, especially when compared with the often trivial nature of the scratch.

Primary syphilis is accompanied by regional lymphadenopathy.

Infectious mononucleosis (glandular fever), caused by the Epstein–Barr virus, mainly affects young adults, producing generalised enlargement of lymphoid tissue including cervical nodes and spleen. Signs and symptoms include fever, headache, malaise, sore throat, skin rash, oral ulceration and petechial haemorrhages of palatal mucosa. Diagnosis includes a positive *Paul–Bunnell* haemagglutinin test and a raised white cell count $(10–20 \times 10^9/l)$ due mainly to an absolute lymphocytosis, with enlarged, abnormal lymphocytes in peripheral blood and lymphoid tissue.

In *measles*, multinucleated (Warthin–Finkeldy) giant cells are present within germinal centres of lymphoid follicles.

Herpetic gingivostomatitis (Chapter 15) is accompanied by painful cervical node enlargement.

In acquired *toxoplasmosis* (Chapter 5), cervical lymphadenopathy is common. Because it is very difficult to demonstrate the causative agent in lymph node sections, diagnosis is confirmed serologically.

Sarcoidosis

Sarcoidosis is a granulomatous inflammation of uncertain aetiology, although a combined infective and immunological basis is probably responsible. It affects many body tissues, including lymph nodes, lung and skin; oral mucosa and salivary glands are much less commonly involved. The characteristic histological feature is non-caseating, granulomatous inflammation containing well-demarcated groups of large, pale-staining ('epithelioid') histiocytes and multinucleated giant cells. There may also be pulmonary fibrosis and hilar node enlargement (detectable radiologically), abnormalities of calcium metabolism with hypercalcaemia and renal calcification, and blindness due to uveal tract involvement. Diagnosis is on clinical grounds, including a positive Kveim test in which intradermal injection of sterile sarcoid

material produces granulomatous inflammation several weeks later. A similar but localised *sarcoid reaction* can be seen in tissues, including lymph nodes, following entry of beryllium or zirconium; it is distinct from, and does not progress to, sarcoidosis.

Neoplasms

Neoplastic cells in lymph nodes are mainly metastatic via lymph from non-lymphoid tissues. The remainder arise from lymphoid cells and are lymphomas.

Metastatic (secondary) deposits

These are commonly found in regional lymph nodes draining the site of the primary tumour, although eventually lymphatic and haematogenous spread can lead to widespread metastatic disease. Although lymphatic spread is most often associated with carcinomas, it can also occur in sarcomas. Enlarged nodes adjacent to malignant neoplasms are likely to be firm and, histologically, to show non-specific, reactive changes with or without tumour deposits; if extensively involved, the normal architecture is completely destroyed.

Lymphomas

Lymphomas are primary neoplasms of extramedullary lymphoreticular tissues. Classifications are extremely complicated, as they include neoplasms of varying behaviour, morphology and prognosis; furthermore, distinctions between lymphomas and leukaemias (Chapter 20) may be blurred (e.g. well-differentiated lymphocytic lymphoma may precede chronic lymphocytic leukaemia). When considering lymphomas, Hodgkin's disease is treated as a separate group of conditions, on clinical and histological grounds, from non-Hodgkin's lymphoma (Table 21.1). Most lymphomas arise within lymph nodes; extranodal lymphomas are mentioned separately later.

Hodgkin's disease. This is the commonest lymphoma; it usually affects young or old adults, and begins as painless lymphadenopathy. Patients may also have a low grade periodic (Pel–Ebstein) fever, anaemia and immunological abnormalities

Table 21.1 Classification of lymphomas

Hodgkin's disease—
    Lymphocyte predominant
    Nodular sclerosing
    Mixed cellularity
    Lymphocyte depleted

Non-Hodgkin's lymphoma—
    Nodular lymphoma:
        Lymphocytic (poorly differentiated)
        Mixed (lymphocytic and histiocytic)
        Histiocytic
    Diffuse lymphoma:
        Lymphocytic (well or poorly differentiated)
        Mixed (lymphocytic and histiocytic)
        Histiocytic
        Undifferentiated (Burkitt type)
        Undifferentiated (non-Burkitt type)

Extranodal Lymphoma

allowing recurrent viral, fungal and protozoal infections. Histologically, the pathognomonic feature is the *Reed–Sternberg cell*, a large, usually binucleate cell with 'mirror-image' nuclei; it is probably the neoplastic cell, but its precise origin is still unknown. The different histological types reflect disease progression and the balance between defence cells and neoplastic cells.

In the *lymphocyte predominant* form, the affected node is replaced by mature lymphocytes and histiocytes, and there are few Reed–Sternberg cells.

The *nodular sclerosing* type is characterised by a thickened fibrous capsule with collagen bands passing towards the centre of the node and by vacuolated Reed–Sternberg cells (*lacunar cells*).

The *mixed cellularity* type shows numerous Reed–Sternberg cells and an infiltrate of eosinophils, neutrophils, plasma cells, lymphocytes and histiocytes.

In the *lymphocyte depleted* form, numerous Reed–Sternberg cells are present, lymphocytes are few and some fibrosis is common.

Affected nodes are rubbery, but become bound together and firm; as the disease progresses, tumour deposits may be found in spleen, liver, bone marrow and other tissues. It is important, for the correct choice of treatment, that extent of disease is determined when the condition is first diagnosed, as this, together with histological type and vascular invasion, influences prognosis. Thus, as well as lymph node biopsies, bone marrow

examination, splenectomy and liver biopsies are routinely performed. Prognosis is best when the disease is confined to a single group of nodes (stage I) and is lymphocyte predominant; widespread involvement of non-lymphoid tissues (stage IV), lymphocyte-depleted histology and vascular invasion indicate a much poorer prognosis. With the exception of the nodular sclerosing type, which tends to remain as such, the disease gradually progresses from lymphocyte predominant to lymphocyte depleted; this progression accelerates as the disease worsens, and death may occur within weeks or months if diagnosis is made at the lymphocyte-depleted phase. Overall, with treatment, over 60% of patients survive 10 years.

Non-Hodgkin's lymphoma. This arises mainly in lymph nodes, and most are B cell in origin. Classifications here are still evolving, and that listed in Table 21.1 is but one of many.

Nodular (follicular) lymphomas mainly affect elderly patients. The normal lymph node architecture is effaced and replaced by lymphoid nodules ('follicles') containing neoplastic cells, either poorly differentiated lymphocytes, histiocytes or both. They generally have a better prognosis than their diffuse counterparts but, with time, many progress to diffuse lymphomas.

In *diffuse lymphomas*, the node is replaced by sheets of neoplastic cells. They spread early via lymphatics to other lymphoid and non-lymphoid tissues, and thus are often diagnosed late; accordingly, 5-year survival is approximately 25%.

One form of diffuse lymphoma, the *Burkitt lymphoma*, has a good prognosis. It is the commonest childhood malignancy in East Africa, and has also been diagnosed in the USA and Europe. The African type is thought to be caused by Epstein Barr virus infection in patients with immunological abnormalities caused by malaria. If untreated, it is rapidly fatal, but it responds extremely well to cytotoxic drug therapy. It is frequently multifocal and extranodal, involving jaw bones, abdominal viscera, thyroid and salivary glands, but can arise in many other sites. The typical histological appearance is of macrophages scattered in a background of small round neoplastic cells, producing a 'starry sky' appearance.

Extranodal lymphomas. These account for a variable, but significant, proportion of lymphomas

(24% in the USA). Most occur in the elderly, typically in upper respiratory and gastrointestinal tracts, as well as skin, bone, salivary glands and lung. Nearly all are diffuse rather than nodular, and of lymphocytic or histiocytic types. In contrast, only 5% of Hodgkin's disease begins extranodally.

SPLEEN

Normal

From the capsule, fibrous trabecula extend towards the centre, carrying blood vessels which permeate the organ as sinusoids. The *white pulp* is lymphoid tissue, surrounding smaller arteries as round Malpighian corpuscles (*bodies*), which frequently contain germinal centres; the *red pulp*, sinusoids and macrophages, occupies the remainder of the organ. Although not essential to life, the spleen has several functions, including immunological reactions by white pulp cells, phagocytosis of circulating microorganisms, removal of old or damaged red blood cells by macrophages and destruction of platelets and leucocytes.

Splenomegaly

Splenomegaly—significant splenic enlargement— can have many causes, and is due to an increase in white pulp, red pulp or both.

Infection by pyogenic organisms in septicaemia leads to enlargement, vascular congestion and polymorph accumulation; abscess formation is, however, uncommon. Non-pyogenic bacterial infections (e.g. typhoid, brucellosis and miliary tuberculosis) may also produce enlargement, as may infectious mononucleosis and malaria.

Haematological causes include enhanced red cell phagocytosis and breakdown (e.g. in haemolytic anaemias and polycythaemia) and extramedullary haemopoiesis (Chapter 20).

In *portal hypertension*, the spleen is enlarged, congested and even fibrotic (Chapter 17).

Amyloidosis produces, in addition to generalised red pulp involvement, the 'sago spleen' in which enlarged and translucent Malpighian corpuscles are prominent against the red pulp background.

Neoplasms

Neoplasms are usually leukaemias and lymphomas. Secondary deposits are uncommon, and are more often from sarcomas than carcinomas.

THYMUS

Normal

The thymus is a poorly understood organ in the anterior mediastinum; its main role is T lymphocyte production (Chapter 6). It reaches its maximum size in childhood, and involutes in adolescence.

Both lobes contain numerous lobules each with a peripheral *cortex* surrounding a central *medulla*. The cortex lacks lymphoid follicles and germinal centres, and consists of sheets of small lymphocytes; the medulla contains *Hassall's corpuscles*, accumulations of concentric epithelial cells.

Failure of development results in primary *T cell immunodeficiencies* such as Di George's syndrome and combined immunological deficiency (Chapter 6); hyperplasia and neoplasia can also lead to immunological abnormalities, including myasthenia gravis (Chapter 23).

Neoplasms

Primary neoplasms are rare.

The *benign thymoma* is the commonest; it arises from epithelial cells but contains a variable proportion of lymphocytes. It is often symptomless, but can produce pressure effects on oesophagus, trachea and superior vena cava, and may be associated with immunologically related diseases (e.g. myasthenia gravis and, very rarely, systemic lupus erythematosus).

Lymphomas are even less common. One, the *Sternberg tumour*, is likely to progress to acute lymphoblastic leukaemia in children.

22

Bone diseases

Normal
Developmental abnormalities
Fractures
Types
Healing
Complications

Infection
Osteomyelitis
Tuberculosis
Syphilis
Metabolic disorders
Osteoporosis

Vitamin D deficiency
Paget's disease
Neoplasms
Benign
Malignant
Metastatic

Normal

Bone is a connective tissue containing a collagen matrix (*osteoid*) on which calcium salts are deposited. When first synthesised by *osteocytes*, collagen fibres of osteoid are irregularly distributed, and when calcified produce *woven bone*; subsequent gradual remodelling produces *lamellar bone*, so called because its collagen bundles are arranged concentrically. In adults, woven bone is seen only when new bone is being produced rapidly (e.g. in fracture callus, Paget's disease and hyperparathyroidism). Mature lamellar bone is constantly being remodelled by resorption (mainly by *osteoclasts*, with the scalloped edges known as *Howship's lacunae*) and continued deposition and calcification of osteoid.

Outer, *cortical bone* is dense, whereas the more central *cancellous bone* contains numerous trabecula separated by bone marrow. In adults, unmineralized osteoid normally covers $13 \pm 7\%$ of trabecular bone surfaces, and each osteoid seam contains one to four collagen bundles arranged as lamellae. Mineralisation of osteoid lags behind its deposition by 6–12 days.

Lamellar bone contains *Haversian systems*, in which a central canal containing blood vessels is surrounded by bone containing osteocytes in lacunae.

DEVELOPMENTAL ABNORMALITIES

Achondroplasia is an inherited dwarfism with defective endochondral ossification; intramembranous bone formation is normal. Affected individuals have shortened limbs, hands and feet, and the middle third of the face is underdeveloped, producing malocclusion.

Osteogenesis imperfecta is an inherited collagen abnormality producing weak, fragile bones. Bony trabecula are greatly reduced in number; bones therefore fracture easily, but they do heal, even though eventually they may become deformed. Deafness from otosclerosis and blue eye sclera are also part of the condition. Abnormal tooth development (including discoloured and poorly formed dentine, pulp chamber obliteration and root fractures) affects both deciduous and permanent dentitions (80% and 35% of patients respectively).

Osteopetrosis (Albers–Schönberg disease) is an hereditary condition leading to increased bone density and decreased marrow spaces. Cranial nerve compression and bone fractures occur.

Cherubism, an autosomal dominant, causes bilateral jaw swellings in childhood. Progressive jaw enlargement, orbital floor involvement and upward eye displacement produce the cherubic appearance. Affected bones are replaced by fibrous tissue containing giant cells resembling osteoclasts. Tooth eruption is abnormal and deciduous teeth are shed early. However, the condition invariably stabilises and often regresses at puberty.

Fibrous dysplasia represents arrest of bone development at the woven bone stage. It affects one or many bones (monostotic or polyostotic respectively), and is more common in females; sometimes it is accompanied by melanin (café-au-lait) skin pigmentation and sexual precocity—*Albright's syndrome*. Jaw involvement occurs in

20% of polyostotic cases. Affected bones show progressive swelling in childhood or early adulthood, but growth does eventually cease. Histologically, bone is replaced by cellular fibrous tissue containing thinned trabecula, and the abnormal area blends imperceptibly with unaffected bone (cf. ossifying fibroma). Sometimes, bone enlargement is considerable, and surgical treatment may be necessary.

FRACTURES

Types

Greenstick fractures are typically seen in children whose bones are protected by a thick periosteum. The periosteum is not torn, the bone is not displaced and healing is rapid.

Simple fractures extend through bone and periosteum into soft tissues but do not communicate with the exterior or any internal body surface.

Compound fractures communicate with a body surface, external or internal. Examples include jaw fractures breaching the oral mucosa.

Spontaneous fractures are due to abnormal muscular forces.

Pathological fractures occur when bone, weakened by disease (e.g. neoplasms and osteogenesis imperfecta), is unable to withstand normal forces.

In *comminuted fractures*, bone is shattered into several fragments.

Healing

Fracture healing is similar to that already outlined for skin wounds (Chapter 4). Haemorrhage from torn blood vessels occurs at the fracture site and may extend into surrounding soft tissues. This stimulates acute inflammation followed by osteoclastic removal of devitalised tissue fragments and adjacent intact bone at the fracture ends. As the fibrin clot is removed by macrophages, it becomes replaced by granulation tissue, the vascular component of which is derived from periosteal and endosteal capillaries. Osteoblasts differentiate from the periosteal layer and endosteal marrow spaces; the former deposit osteoid peripherally around the fracture site at right angles to the bone axis so that a fusiform mass forms across the bone

ends, while the latter gradually obliterate the endosteal gap with osteoid. During this process, osteoid, which subsequently mineralises to form woven bone, may be deposited on the surface of necrotic bone fragments; only with time and continued remodelling will this non-vital bone be replaced. The term *callus* describes the woven bone mass uniting the fractured bone ends. It is subsequently remodelled to form lamellar (including both cortical and medullary) bone, this process being aided by progressive functional demands placed on it. An adequate blood supply is of great importance in fracture healing—*avascular necrosis* results if the blood supply is severely impaired. This often affects the femoral head in femoral neck fractures, where the end artery is damaged; it may also follow vessel blockage in sickle cell anaemia and irradiation. Extensive mandibular necrosis in the elderly may follow periosteal elevation, as gradual reduction in blood flow through the inferior dental artery is a recognised age change. A diminished blood supply or failure to immobilise bone ends may cause cartilage formation at the fracture site; endochondral ossification may allow subsequent conversion to bone.

Complications of fracture healing

Non-union (failure of bone ends to unite) follows severe bone loss and occurs when soft tissues (e.g. muscle) become interposed. Each bone end becomes rounded and undergoes 'healing' but without bony continuity.

Delayed union may follow impairment of blood supply, excessive local haemorrhage (e.g. in haemophilia), inadequate immobilisation, local infection or generalised deficiency states (e.g. of protein, vitamin C or vitamin D). Healing takes longer in old age due to a reduction in general body metabolism. To promote healing, splinting is used to immobilise bone ends. Fractured ribs often develop cartilaginous and fibrous tissues at fracture sites as they cannot be immobilised without interfering significantly with respiration; if movement of bone ends is excessive, a false joint may be created.

Healing of extraction sockets involves principles of fracture and skin wound healing. Haemorrhage following extraction is sometimes considerable, but it is remarkable how efficient healing is when considering the extensive surface area of bone exposed during multiple extractions (frequently, the buccal plate is fractured and either displaced laterally or removed with the tooth if fused) and the probability of salivary contamination. Usually healing is uneventful, but sometimes, the initial blood clot breaks down and the infected socket becomes painful (*dry socket*); this generally follows either excessive haemorrhage (e.g. in the vascular phase of Paget's disease and haemophilia) or inadequate bleeding into the socket (e.g. in the sclerotic phase of Paget's disease). Once healing is complete, there is slow continued loss of the now non-functional alveolar bone over many years.

INFECTIONS

Osteomyelitis

Osteomyelitis (inflammation of bone) is usually due to infection; *periostitis* indicates involvement of subperiosteal bone.

Acute osteomyelitis was a serious condition, but is rarely seen nowadays thanks to advances in surgical techniques and antibiotics. Typically, it affects long bones of children, and follows bacteraemia from a distant focus of infection (e.g. a boil), organisms settling in an area of damaged, usually traumatised bone. Other routes of organism entry include direct spread (e.g. after dental extractions and via necrotic root canals following dental caries) and compound fractures. *Staphylococcus aureus* is the commonest causative organism, although streptococci, *Haemophilus influenzae* and others are less commonly implicated; *Salmonella osteomyelitis* may complicate sickle cell anaemia.

Extensive suppuration spreads through the marrow cavity and erodes the cortex to spread over the bone surface below the loosely attached periosteum. Thrombosis of local blood vessels is common, and causes bone death. Resorption takes place at the junction of dead and vital bone so that a *sequestrum* of smooth, dead bone becomes detached. From the undersurface of the raised periosteum, new bone is formed and may encircle the dead shaft of a long bone as an *involucrum*. Gaps (*cloacae*) in the involucrum provide a passage

for small pieces of necrotic bone (sequestra) and pus to track outwards to discharge on to body surfaces.

Complications include joint involvement (*septic arthritis*) and, in children, damage to the epiphyseal plate with *growth disturbances. Septicaemia* may lead to widespread systemic abscesses. Adults are much less prone to develop typical acute osteomyelitis as the tightly bound periosteum is perforated rather than lifted by pus. When the osteomyelitis is less severe, or where antibiotics have been used inappropriately, a localised abscess (*Brodie's abscess*) may develop. When teeth are extracted from a jaw in which the blood supply is impaired (e.g. after irradiation for malignancy), there is a risk of rapidly spreading infection (radiation-induced osteomyelitis or *osteoradionecrosis*, Chapter 11).

Chronic osteomyelitis is common in the jaws, and follows infection from non-vital pulps of teeth. Adjacent bone may be occupied by inflamed granulation tissue or, if tissue resistance is good, there may be bone sclerosis. A similar condition is seen in long bones and jaws of young patients as *chronic osteomyelitis with proliferative periostitis (Garré's sclerosing osteomyelitis)*, in which periosteal reaction to infection produces bony swelling.

Tuberculosis

Tuberculosis is much less common since the advent of effective antibiotics. It can affect most bones, including the mandible, although vertebrae, hands, feet and long bones are more often involved; it follows haematogenous spread from a pre-existing focus, usually in the lung. Caseous necrosis leads to slow destruction of bony trabecula; with vertebral involvement, there may be anterior collapse, spinal cord compression and neurological symptoms.

Syphilis

Syphilis may be *congenital*, affecting the metaphysis (*osteochondritis*) with possible epiphyseal separation and growth retardation; the depressed, *saddle nose* is caused by destruction of the nasal septum. *Acquired syphilis*, usually tertiary, may produce periostitis and bone destruction with sequestration (*gummas*) anywhere, including palate and skull; endarteritis is important in gumma formation.

METABOLIC DISORDERS

Osteoporosis

Osteoporosis is a reduction in density and amount of trabecular bone due to an imbalance between deposition and resorption, mineralisation being normal. Involving women more often than men, it may be *idiopathic* (representing an exaggerated age change) or *secondary*, including the commonest variety, *postmenopausal*, as well as *inadequate collagen synthesis* (e.g. vitamin C and protein deficiency), *endocrine abnormalities* (e.g. Cushing's syndrome and thyrotoxicosis) and *immobilisation* producing disuse atrophy (e.g. prolonged bed rest and paralysis). Bones are softer and fracture more easily than normal; vertebral collapse with anterior bowing of the spine is common, causing pain and loss of height. Jaw involvement may be evident radiographically as a generalised radiolucency.

Vitamin D deficiency

Vitamin D and calcium metabolism are considered in Chapter 19. Vitamin D deficiency (or insensitivity to its action) results in softened bones due to defective osteoid mineralisation. Thus, trabecular surfaces are covered with a greater proportion of osteoid, each osteoid seam being thicker than normal. Even when mineralisation does occur, it is at a reduced rate. In children, *rickets* results and in adults, *osteomalacia*. Both are usually due either to dietary vitamin D deficiency or to lack of the sunlight required for its synthesis in skin. Serum calcium and phosphate levels are lowered and alkaline phosphatase is raised; hyperparathyroidism may develop in an attempt to restore the serum calcium.

In *rickets*, inadequate mineralisation interferes with endochondral ossification; epiphyses are enlarged and prominent as cartilage cells continue to be produced—in costochondral junctions this produces the typical '*rickety rosary*' and *pigeon chest*. Bones fracture easily; skull bones are soft; legs become bowed and often knock-kneed (*coxa vara*) and there is muscle weakness. Vitamin D

therapy does not overcome permanent deformities but does permit adequate mineralisation to proceed.

Causes of *osteomalacia* also include malabsorption, partial gastrectomy and chronic renal failure. The main effect is weakened bones with an increased tendency to fracture. Defects of mineralisation during tooth formation in children may sometimes cause enamel hypoplasia, and frequently there is an increase in interglobular dentine and impaired tooth eruption. In hypophosphataemic vitamin-D-resistant rickets (an inherited renal tubular phosphate reabsorption defect), there is also pulp enlargement extending in places to the amelodentinal junction, with the risk of pulp exposure and periapical abscesses in caries-free teeth.

PAGET'S DISEASE

Paget's disease of bone is of unknown aetiology, although a slow virus may contribute. It usually affects the middle aged and elderly, men more than women, and mainly those of Anglo–Saxon descent. Vertebrae, skull and pelvis are often involved, but sometimes only one bone is affected. Initially, there is increased bone resorption by enlarged osteoclasts and increased vascularity; radiographically this produces radiolucency (*osteoporosis circumscripta*). Subsequently, osteoblastic activity is intense, and bone turnover is greatly increased until eventually dense, poorly vascular bone is found (hence the 'cotton-wool' appearance on radiographs). Maxillary bones may enlarge to produce 'leonine facies'; the patient may complain that dentures or a hat no longer fit, and long bones may become enlarged and bowed (e.g. sabre tibias). Enhanced bone turnvover is detected by an increase in urinary hydroxyproline and serum alkaline phosphatase; microscopically there is a '*mosaic appearance*' of irregular jigsaw-like, interdigitating cement lines. Serum calcium and phosphate are normal. Other clinical features include neurological symptoms (e.g. deafness and spinal root problems due to nerve compression by bone enlargement) and drifting of teeth.

Complications include bone fractures, high output cardiac failure due to increased bone vascularity, osteo-arthrosis from abnormal stresses on joints and an increased risk of osteogenic sarcoma or giant cell tumour of bone.

Dental complications are haemorrhage on tooth extraction, socket infection and osteomyelitis, an increased risk of jaw fracture and ankylosis between cementum and alveolar bone.

NEOPLASMS

Benign neoplasms of cartilage

Osteocartilaginous exostosis (osteochondroma) accounts for 60%, and presents as a mass growing outwards from the surface, usually of long bones, hands or feet. It affects children, and consists of a cartilage cap undergoing endochondral ossification. It will recur if inadequately excised. Malignant change is rare in solitary lesions, but if multiple, a chondrosarcoma will ultimately develop in up to 20% of patients.

Enchondromas are within the medullary cavity. In hands and feet, the commonest sites, they are benign, but in long bones they may become malignant. Multiple enchondromas (Ollier's disease) become malignant in up to 50% of cases. In *Maffucci's syndrome* they may be associated with haemangiomas in soft tissues.

Benign neoplasms of bone

Osteoid osteoma is usually under 1 cm diameter, and consists of a central vascular nidus of osteoblastic tissue surrounded by a comparatively radiolucent zone and with a peripheral rim of sclerotic bone.

The *benign osteoblastoma* has a similar appearance, but is larger, more frequently painful, and lacks the central nidus. It consists of active osteoblastic tissue in a vascular stroma.

Ossifying fibroma is often confused with fibrous dysplasia (see above). Both comprise cellular fibrous tissue containing a few trabecula and both can involve jaws. However, ossifying fibroma is seen in patients over the age of 20 years, and is delineated from unaffected bone both radiographically and histologically by a rim of fibrous tissue.

Giant cell tumour (*osteoclastoma*) usually develops at the ends of long bones in young adults, and

only appears in jaws as a complication of Paget's disease. It comprises very large multinucleated giant cells in a fibrous tissue stroma. Pain, swelling and pathological fractures can be presenting symptoms. Although most follow a benign course, some recur, and 15–30% may ultimately metastasise. Generally, those with cytological evidence of malignancy behave badly.

Malignant neoplasms of cartilage and bone

Chondrosarcoma develops in adults, usually males, either de novo or from pre-existing benign tumours. Overall, it is slightly less frequent than osteogenic sarcoma; in the jaws where, unlike elsewhere, cartilaginous neoplasms are much more likely to be malignant than benign, it is uncommon. Pain and swelling occur, but growth is generally slow, and local spread and metastases may take many years to develop. Histologically, there may be obvious cytological evidence of malignancy, but sometimes this may be slight, making true diagnosis very difficult.

Osteogenic sarcoma (osteosarcoma) incorporates osteoid production by malignant cells. Unlike chondrosarcoma, it frequently affects children or young adults, although a few cases follow irradiation or Paget's disease. Males are affected more than females, and the commonest site is around the knee. Local swelling and spread may be rapid; blood stream dissemination takes place early, often to lungs, so the 5-year survival is only 10–20%. Jaw lesions usually develop in middle age and have a 5-year survival of 20–35%.

Ewing's tumour is an uncommon malignant neoplasm of uncertain histogenesis which affects long bones in childhood and early adulthood. Histologically, it consists of sheets of small, round cells containing glycogen. Pain is usually a feature, often with anaemia and fever. Metastases are common, particularly to other bones and lungs. The disease progresses rapidly and has a poor prognosis, 5-year survival being 10–30%.

Histiocytosis X is a triad of related but uncommon conditions where the main cell type appears to be the histiocyte. *Eosinophilic granuloma of bone* affects children, usually 5–10 years old. One or occasionally more bones (skull, jaws, long bones) may be involved; there is a circumscribed radiolucency comprising eosinophil poly-morphs and histiocytes. Prognosis is good. *Hand–Schüller–Christian disease* also affects children, but involves numerous bones, skin, liver, lymph nodes, spleen and lungs. Radiographically, affected bones show 'punched-out' areas. Prognosis is poor, death ultimately occurring after several years. *Letterer–Siwe disease* affects infants and is usually rapidly fatal. There is widespread involvement of soft tissues and bones by sheets of histiocytes.

Primary lymphomas of bone are uncommon and frequently histiocytic (Chapter 21).

Metastatic neoplasms

Metastatic neoplasms are much more common than primary bone tumours. They may originate from many sites, but most arise in prostate, bronchus or breast. Most cause local bone destruction (i.e. are *osteolytic*), and may produce pathological fractures; a few (e.g. prostatic carcinoma) stimulate new bone deposition (i.e. are *osteosclerotic*). Extensive deposits with marrow destruction may result in anemia.

23

Joint, muscle and connective tissue diseases

Joints
Normal
Inflammation
Osteoarthritis
Tumours
Skeletal muscle
Normal

Inflammation
Atrophy
Muscular dystrophies
Myasthenia gravis
Connective tissue diseases
Introduction
Rheumatoid arthritis

Systemic lupus erythematosus
Progressive systemic sclerosis
Dermatomyositis
Rheumatic fever
Polyarteritis nodosa
Dental aspects
Temporomandibular joint

JOINTS

Normal

Most are synovial. The bone ends are covered by a thin, smooth, avascular layer of *articular cartilage* (chondrocytes and matrix); the joint contains rather viscous *synovial fluid* (for lubrication) secreted by the vascular *synovial membrane* lining the cavity and adjacent tendon sheaths. Some are partially or completely divided by fibrocartilagenous *articular discs (menisci)*.

Inflammation

Arthritis may be due to specific infecting agents or of unknown aetiology.

Acute arthritis is usually a complication of septicaemia from a primary focus elsewhere, but widespread antibiotic usage has markedly reduced its incidence. Many organisms may be responsible, particularly staphylococci, streptococci and gonococci. One or more large joints are usually affected, with typical macroscopic and microscopic features of acute inflammation—swelling, redness, excess heat, pain and synovial polymorph infiltration, with pus and fibrin in the joint cavity. Resolution may occur with early treatment, but the acute inflammation rapidly destroys articular cartilage; healing then is by granulation tissue and fibrosis, which ultimately replaces much of the joint cavity, and produces a fibrous union between bone ends (*fibrous ankylosis*) with considerable residual disability.

Tuberculous arthritis is also decreasing in incidence. It may follow bacteraemia (e.g. hip and knee), but may represent direct spread from adjacent bone (e.g. spine—Chapter 22). The synovial membrane is congested and thickened, and tuberculous granulation tissue grows over, destroys and gradually replaces articular cartilage. Early adequate treatment may result in little residual damage, but healing by fibrosis produces progressive ankylosis with deformity and disability.

Rheumatoid arthritis is the commonest inflammatory joint disease in this country. Aetiology is unknown, but it is usually classified as one of the connective tissue diseases (see below).

Ankylosing spondylitis is an inflammatory disease of spinal joints which progresses to ossification (*bony ankylosis*); spinal ligaments and intervertebral disc margins also ossify, and the result is a deformed and rigid spine. It is rare, and usually starts in young males between 15 and 35 years of age; aetiology is unknown, but there may be a genetic predisposition through the HLA system via B27 (Chapter 6). The early synovial changes are those of rheumatoid arthritis.

Gout, discussed in Chapter 7, reflects abnormal purine metabolism, with sodium biurate crystal deposition in many tissues including smaller joints. It may be acute (where the big toe is classically affected and extremely painful) or chronic (with crystals aggregated as tophi). The crystals elicit acute and/or chronic inflammation, with degeneration and destruction of articular cartilage; healing is by fibrosis, with consequent deformity and disability.

Osteoarthritis

Primary osteoarthritis (osteoarthrosis) is degenerative rather than inflammatory. Although it may develop in younger people after previous damage, it usually arises spontaneously in the elderly. Aetiology remains unknown, although functional changes in cartilage are implicated. It is extremely common in both sexes, and mainly affects larger, load-bearing joints (e.g. hip and knee). Initial changes are thinning and splitting (*fibrillation*) of articular cartilage; later, the cartilage disappears, and underlying subchondral bone becomes thickened and smooth (*eburnation*—i.e. like ebony), with irregular outgrowths beyond articular margins (*osteophytes*). Later still, bone remodelling alters considerably the overall shape of joint surfaces. Onset is insidious, and the disease is progressive; affected joints are painful and stiff. No specific treatment is available, and ultimately, surgical replacement may be necessary. Sometimes these patients also develop small bony outgrowths from the dorsal aspect of the terminal phalanges of their fingers (*Heberden's nodes*); there is usually considerable deformity but little local disability.

Secondary osteoarthritis follows pre-existing joint damage. Examples include acute or chronic *traumatic arthritis* (the latter is represented by shoulder disease in workers using pneumatic road drills); irritation by loose bodies (e.g. cartilage or bone fragments) within the joint cavity which interfere with normal function; *neurotrophic joint disease* (such as in syphilis and diabetes mellitus), where loss of nerve function allows painless over-stressing; and following inflammatory disease with damage to articulating surfaces, including gout and chondrocalcinosis (pyrophosphate crystals). Histologically, the changes are as in primary osteoarthritis, but evidence of the predisposing factor(s) may also be present.

Tumours

Bone and cartilage tumours are considered in Chapter 22; neoplasms arising in and immediately around joints are rare, and usually synovial in origin.

Benign synovioma may arise at any adult age, and invariably affects fingers. They are round, firm, lobulated masses composed of regular mononuclear synovial-like cells admixed with multinucleate giant cells. They grow slowly and tend to recur, probably because of inadequate, incomplete initial resection.

Pigmented villonodular synovitis is probably reactive rather than neoplastic. It is usually found in middle-aged males, often in knee or hip joints. The synovium is hyperplastic, and presents a characteristic villous appearance with more solid nodular areas; abundant haemosiderin provides the pigment and imparts a red-brown colour. Although recurrence following excision is frequent, extra-articular spread does not occur.

Synovial sarcoma (*malignant synovioma*) usually arises around hip, knee or ankle in young adults. Local invasion is often extensive, and metastases, particularly haematogenous, tend to occur early. The histological picture is very variable, with spindle cells and cleft-like spaces, and correlates with an equally variable prognosis.

SKELETAL MUSCLE

Normal

Skeletal muscle consists of numerous individual elongated muscle cells or fibres (*myocytes*), with cytoplasm containing many *myofibrils* of interdigitating *myosin* and *actin* filaments which provide characteristic cross-striations. Every fibre is surrounded by a very thin *endomysial sheath*; groups of fibres (*muscle bundles*) are surrounded by a fibrous *perimysium*; an *epimysium* envelops the whole muscle. Each fibre has its own nerve supply, which enters near its midpoint at the *neuromuscular junction* (*motor end plate*); muscle bundles are usually innervated by a single anterior horn cell, and together they form the *motor unit*.

Inflammation

Myositis is uncommon, and usually represents extension from adjacent infective foci (e.g. bones and joints); occasionally it occurs in septicaemia or pyaemia. Changes are variable, but often include muscle necrosis and acute inflammation.

Gas gangrene is a specific infection by anaerobic, spore-bearing organisms, usually *Clostridium welchii* (Chapter 2). They synthesise exotoxins and proteolytic enzymes which produce local muscle fibre necrosis or degeneration and initiate acute inflammation.

Polymyositis is a rare, rapidly progressive connective tissue disease; skin involvement is usual, producing dermatomyositis (see below).

Myositis ossificans usually develops in adolescents or young adults, and often follows trauma. Intra-muscular haemorrhage is followed by organisation into fibrous tissue which is subsequently converted into cartilage and bone, probably by metaplasia. There is local swelling, but it is benign.

Atrophy

Atrophy is loss of muscle fibre bulk, often with replacement fibrosis. It occurs with prolonged disuse and ischaemia, and, to some extent, is common in old age. *Neurogenic atrophy* is secondary to any lower motor neurone disorder (e.g. poliomyelitis, Chapter 24). Affected fibres are reduced in size; initially, they retain their cross-striations, but ultimately disappear to be replaced by fibrous tissue. In neurogenic atrophy, changes are confined to denervated fibres; adjacent innervated fibres remain normal.

Muscular dystrophies

Muscular dystrophies are primary degenerative diseases. Several clinical syndromes exist (e.g. Duchenne), reflecting different muscle distri-butions; aetiology is unknown, but most are heredi-tary and some are X linked. Muscle fibres are affected individually, producing a mixture of normal, degenerate, atrophic and necrotic cells; fat may appear between affected fibres, but inflammation is usually absent. Onset is invariably insidious, progression is almost inevitable, and life expectancy is reduced, often considerably.

Myasthenia gravis

Myasthenia gravis is characterised by muscular weakness, particularly during repeated use, and is due to autoantibodies against acetylcholine receptor sites in neuromuscular junctions. It usually begins in early adult life, and is commoner in women; it follows a very variable course, with marked variations in severity. Muscular changes are often mild, focal and non-specific, and include atrophy, necrosis and chronic inflammation; motor end plates may be irregularly distorted. Associated thymic abnormalities are usual—about 80% show marked hyperplasia and almost 10%

have thymomas (Chapter 21); some improvement often follows thymectomy.

CONNECTIVE TISSUE DISEASES

Introduction

This is a rather vague term incorporating several multisystem diseases, most of which are commoner in females, with certain similar aetiological, patho-logical and clinical features; overlap between diseases may occur. They are sometimes even more vaguely referred to as *rheumatic diseases*, and were formally designated *collagen diseases*, as collagen degeneration and necrosis were thought to be the basic structural changes. Many are as-sociated with autoantibody production, and most have common histological appearances, including acute and chronic inflammation, fibrinoid necrosis and necrotising arteritis.

Rheumatoid arthritis

Rheumatoid arthritis is the commonest, affecting, to some extent, almost 2% of the population in this country. It often develops in females (F:M ratio about 3:1) in early or middle adult life, and, although any synovial joint including the temporo-mandibular may be involved, it usually affects hands and feet most severely. It is seen occasionally in children, usually as severe acute disease (Still's disease).

Aetiology. Most patients have circulating 'rheu-matoid factor'—immune complexes comprising antibody (usually IgM) and antigen (IgG, with the Fc component acting as antigenic determinant). Why these factors develop and how they cause damage remain unknown; joint infection may somehow be involved.

Pathology. In acute attacks or exacerbations, affected joints are swollen, hot and tender, with excess synovial fluid (*synovial effusion*); the synovium shows marked hypertrophy, prolifer-ation, infiltration by polymorphs, lymphocytes and plasma cells and fibrinous exudation. Later, in more chronic cases, articular cartilage is gradually destroyed and replaced by granulation tissue (*pannus*), which subsequently progresses to fibrosis or even ossification (fibrous or bony anky-losis); simultaneously, adjacent ligaments and tendons may be involved, with laxity and deformity, and adjacent muscles become atrophic and wasted. About 20% of cases, usually more severely affected patients, develop subcutaneous *rheumatoid nodules* comprising fibrinoid necrosis surrounded by palisaded (i.e. radially orientated) fibroblasts; occasionally such nodules are found elsewhere (e.g. lung, pleura, pericardium and eyes), and when they develop in lungs of patients with pneumoconiosis it is designated *Caplan's syndrome*. Severe cases sometimes develop a focal necrotising arteritis, and associated thrombosis may produce infarction (e.g. in bowel or myocardium). Long-standing rheumatoid arthritis is now the commonest cause of *secondary amyloidosis* in this country (Chapter 7).

Clinical features. It is a very variable and fluctuating condition, often with a rather insidious onset and frequent remissions. Although corticosteroids and non-steroidal anti-inflammatory drugs may partially suppress and retard joint changes, the disease is usually progressive, with increasing pain, stiffness and deformity; ultimately as ankylosis develops relatively painless, rigid and grossly deformed joints result. Patients may also have Sjögren's syndrome (Chapter 15).

Systemic lupus erythematosus

Systemic lupus erythematosus (SLE) is much less common, and usually affects young women.

Aetiology. Most patients produce autoantibodies to their own nuclear material (particularly deoxyribonuclear protein—*antinuclear factor*); many also have circulating immune complexes (comprising autoantibodies and released nuclear antigens) which elicit type III hypersensitivity reactions (Chapter 6). Reasons why autoantibodies develop are unknown, although a reaction to sunlight or drugs is possible, and an initiating viral infection has been postulated; furthermore, such patients show an increased incidence of HLA-B8. In 70–80% of cases, some peripheral blood polymorphs contain phagocytosed acellular basophilic nuclear material complexed with antinuclear antibody and complement ('*LE cells*'). Adverse drug reactions are common in SLE.

Pathology. Any organ may be involved, but SLE particularly affects kidneys, skin, serosal surfaces (i.e. pleura, pericardium and peritoneum), endocardium, joints and small blood vessels. Renal involvement is very common, and chiefly produces immune-complex-mediated glomerulonephritis (Chapter 18); the skin usually shows an erythematous maculopapular rash, which often presents a characteristic '*butterfly*' distribution across the face; elsewhere, there is fibrinoid necrosis, acute and/or chronic inflammation which may be granulomatous, and subsequent fibrosis; vascular changes often produce ischaemia and infarction.

Clinical features. Onset is usually insidious and remissions may occur. Numerous local and general symptoms are possible; SLE, therefore, may mimic many other diseases. It is overall progressive, and although it may be retarded by corticosteroid therapy prognosis is poor; death is usually from chronic renal failure.

Progressive systemic sclerosis

Progressive systemic sclerosis, sometimes inaccurately called *scleroderma*, is a rare, insidious disease, usually appearing in middle-aged women. It is characterised by arterial and arteriolar intimal thickening and proliferation; consequent luminal narrowing produces ischaemia and progressive fibrosis. Many systems are involved, including skin (which becomes thickened and tense, with limitation of joint movements), cardiac and skeletal muscles (with ischaemia and infarction), oesophagus (causing dysphagia), kidneys (producing renal function impairment and secondary hypertension), lungs (predisposing to infections and fibrosis) and hands (with Raynaud's phenomenon). Aetiology is completely unknown, and no characteristic autoantibodies have been described. Progressive is inevitable but usually very slow, and death may well be due to other, unrelated diseases.

Dermatomyositis

Dermatomyositis is very rare. The skin shows an erythematous rash (cf. SLE); skeletal and cardiac muscles show patchy degeneration and necrosis, with acute and chronic inflammation (*polymyositis*). Onset is usually fairly acute and progression rapid; prognosis is therefore poor.

Rheumatic fever

Rheumatic fever, now uncommon in this country, is often classified as a connective tissue disease. It is discussed in Chapter 13.

Polyarteritis nodosa

Polyarteritis nodosa is also usually considered in this group. It is discussed in Chapter 12.

DENTAL ASPECTS

The temporomandibular joint (TMJ) has a complex pattern of sliding and rotational movements. Its structure is unusual for a synovial joint in that the mandibular condyle has a surface fibrous articulating layer, a deeper cellular or intermediate zone, a cartilage zone and, deepest of all, the bony end plate.

Pain dysfunction syndrome is common, and affects young women. Pain in the TMJ and associated muscles (temporalis, masseter, medial and lateral pterygoids) is worse in the morning and is caused by muscle spasm in an attempt to protect the joint from irregular and premature contacts of opposing teeth. Treatment includes occlusal adjustment to eliminate abnormal contacts. On light microscopy the condyle appears normal, but ultrastructurally shows collagen and fibroblast degeneration of the fibrous articular layer.

Osteoarthritis (osteoarthrosis) of the TMJ is similar to that elsewhere, but with certain clinical and histological differences. It is common in middle age, it affects females much more than males, and approximately half the patients have previously suffered from the pain dysfunction syndrome. Histologically, in addition to loss of fibrous, intermediate and cartilaginous zones, there is early perforation of the subarticular bony end plate, with attempts at repair by growth of fibrous tissue over the damaged areas. Prognosis is quite good, as 50% are pain free after 1 year of conservative, including steroid, treatment; only a small proportion require surgical removal of the condyle.

24

Nervous system diseases

Brain	Raised intracranial pressure	Motor neurone disease	Normal
Normal	Tumours	Tumours	Inflammation
Inflammation	**Spinal cord**	**Peripheral nerves**	Glaucoma
Cerebrovascular disease	Normal	Normal	Cataract
Head injuries	Inflammation	Trauma	Tumours
Hydrocephalus	Spinal cord compression	Peripheral neuropathy	**Dental aspects**
Demyelinating diseases	Syringomyelia	Tumours	Facial paralysis
Degenerative diseases	Subacute combined degeneration	**Eye**	

BRAIN

Normal

The brain lies within the *skull* (*cranial cavity*), and comprises two cerebral hemispheres (*cerebrum*), *cerebellum* and *brain stem* (*midbrain, pons* and *medulla oblongata*).

The brain is enveloped by three membranes (*meninges*). The *dura mater* is thick and inelastic; it acts as internal periosteum to skull bones, and provides septa which partially subdivide the cranial cavity. The *arachnoid* is thinner and more delicate, and separated from the dura by a very narrow, almost potential *subdural space*. The *pia mater* is a very thin, highly vascular membrane, very closely adherent to the brain and separated from the arachnoid by the *subarachnoid space* containing cerebrospinal fluid (CSF) and major cerebral blood vessels.

The brain contains two cell groups. *Neurones* are specialised nerve cells consisting of a nerve cell body, small cytoplasmic processes (*dendrites*) and a longer process surrounded by a myelin sheath (*axon*); most cell bodies and dendrites are found peripherally, and constitute *grey matter*, whilst most axons are deeper and produce *white matter*. *Neuroglia*, the other cell group, provide support, and include *astrocytes* (which produce supportive glial fibrils), *oligodendrocytes* (producing intracerebral myelin), *ependymal cells* (lining the ventricular system) and *microglia* (part of the mononuclear phagocyte system).

Cerebrospinal fluid (CSF) surrounds, supports and protects the brain. It is similar to blood plasma and is secreted into the lateral cerebral ventricles by the *choroid plexuses*. It flows through various foramina, initially into the third ventricle, then the fourth ventricle and finally into the subarachnoid space; from there it is absorbed, mainly by arachnoid granulations, into dural venous sinuses.

Inflammation

Inflammation is invariably due to infection; many organisms may be responsible, and may involve meninges (i.e. *meningitis*) and/or brain substance (*encephalitis*).

Acute bacterial meningitis

Acute bacterial meningitis mainly involves the pia and arachnoid, and organisms proliferate in CSF.

Aetiology. Several bacteria may be responsible, particularly *Neisseria meningitidis* (meningococcus), *Streptococcus pneumoniae* and, especially in infants, *Escherichia coli*; most reach the meninges via the blood stream, although some enter from adjacent structures (e.g. air sinuses and middle ear), particularly when the skull is fractured.

Pathology. Typical acute inflammation is produced, and fibrinous or purulent exudate accumulates in the subarachnoid space, mainly around the base of the brain; organisms and polymorphs are present in the CSF, a small quantity of which may be withdrawn by *lumbar puncture* and examined.

Clinical features. Meningeal irritation (from numerous causes including acute inflammation) causes headache, neck stiffness, confusion and drowsiness. When meningococci are responsible, the bacteraemic phase preceding the meningitis may be associated with a characteristic haemorrhagic rash (hence '*spotted fever*') and occasionally with rapidly fatal, massive bilateral adrenal haemorrhages (*Waterhouse–Friderichsen syndrome*).

Results. Early, appropriate antibiotic treatment may promote resolution; delayed or inadequate treatment will allow some progression to chronic inflammation, with subsequent fibrous meningeal thickening causing obstruction to CSF flow (hydrocephalus—see below) and cranial nerve compression.

Tuberculous meningitis

Tuberculous meningitis is now uncommon, but recently its incidence has started to increase. It is invariably blood borne, usually from primary or secondary pulmonary disease, and may either represent single organ involvement or reflect miliary dissemination. Organisms proliferate in CSF and produce meningeal thickening (by chronic inflammation, fibrosis and tubercle formation) and fibrinous exudation. Onset is usually insidious, with vague clinical symptoms. Without treatment, death is almost inevitable; treatment may halt progression, but fibrous adhesions usually produce CSF blockage and various neurological disturbances.

Bacterial encephalitis

Bacterial encephalitis is usually due to direct extension from acute bacterial or tuberculous meningitis, and is often superficial and relatively mild.

Brain abscesses are now uncommon; many bacteria may be responsible. Organisms arrive either via the blood stream (pyaemia or septic emboli, especially from lungs), when they are often multiple, or by direct spread from an adjacent infected focus (e.g. middle ear and air sinuses, particularly mastoid or following penetrating wounds), when they are often solitary. Sites vary with aetiology—haematogenous abscesses are commonly parietal, whilst middle ear infection produces temporal or cerebellar lesions. There is localised pus formation with brain destruction,

distortion and oedema; adjacent astrocytes produce a glial tissue capsule. Symptoms are often very vague, and may include epilepsy and features of raised intracranial pressure (see below); extension and rupture into the subarachnoid space or a ventricle produces meningitis and is usually fatal.

Viral meningitis

Viral meningitis (*aseptic meningitis*) is common, especially in children; many viruses, including enteroviruses, herpes simplex and mumps, may be responsible, and all gain access via the blood stream during viraemia. Meninges are congested, with marked lymphocytic infiltration, and there are excess lymphocytes in the CSF. Features of meningeal irritation (see above) are present, and usually last 7–10 days. Full recovery is usual; residual complications are uncommon; death is very rare.

Viral encephalitis

Viral encephalitis is rare, but often fatal. In the UK, herpes simplex is the commonest organism, but elsewhere arboviruses may cause epidemics; haematogenous spread is usual. Although macroscopic appearances are often undramatic, nerve cells (in which viral replication occurs) show extensive degeneration, intranuclear inclusions and necrosis, and there is predominantly perivascular infiltration by lymphocytes, plasma cells and macrophages. Clinical features include pyrexia, drowsiness, paralysis and tremors; progressive and fairly rapid deterioration to death usually occurs.

Rabies, although absent from this country, is endemic in many areas, including Europe, India and parts of the Americas. Transmission to humans is via saliva of rabid animals (usually dogs) introduced by bites. The virus reaches the brain along peripheral nerves, the incubation period (usually 1–2 months) depending on the distance between the bite and the brain. The pathology is that of viral encephalitis, and neurones characteristically contain well-defined, intracytoplasmic, eosinophilic inclusions (*Negri bodies*). Clinically, there is usually hyperactivity and marked irritability, with muscular contractions, spasms and convulsions; these typically affect swallowing, and hence cause reluctance to drink (*hydrophobia*). The disease is progressive and invariably fatal.

Syphilis

Syphilis usually affects the brain in the tertiary stage, but may represent congenital disease (Chapter 5).

Meningovascular syphilis occurs relatively early. Meninges are opaque and thickened, especially around the base of the brain, by fibrosis and chronic inflammation; vessels show mural thickening and luminal narrowing by intimal proliferation (*endarteritis obliterans*); *gummas* (as seen elsewhere in tertiary syphilis) may also be present, both in meninges and within the brain. Clinical features may include meningeal irritation (see above), CSF obstruction and hydrocephalus (see below), cranial nerve damage, ischaemia from vascular involvement and raised intracranial pressure (see below) from gummas.

General paralysis of the insane is a later manifestation. It is a chronic, slowly progressive encephalitis with continuing neuronal destruction and replacement by gliosis producing motor, sensory, intellectual and psychiatric disturbances. Progression is inevitable, but may be retarded considerably by appropriate antisyphilitic chemotherapy.

Other infections (see also Chapter 5)

Fungi. Cryptococcus neoformans may cause a chronic meningitis. Others (e.g. *Candida albicans* and *Aspergillus fumigatus*) usually represent opportunistic infections in immunodeficient patients.

Toxoplasmosis. The brain may be involved in both congenital and acquired diseases.

Cerebrovascular disease

Cerebrovascular disease, covering both haemorrhage and infarction, is common, and accounts for about 15% of all deaths in this country. It is often referred to as '*cerebrovascular accident*' (CVA), as clinical differentiation between haemorrhage and infarction is usually extremely difficult, if not impossible.

Spontaneous intracranial haemorrhage

Spontaneous intracranial haemorrhage may be intracerebral or subarachnoid (cf. traumatic haemorrhages—see below).

Intracerebral haemorrhage is usually associated with systemic hypertension (Chapter 12), where multiple tiny microaneurysms develop in small intracerebral arteries, and one or more subsequently rupture. It appears as a large haemorrhage with adjacent brain tissue destruction, the internal capsule and pons being the commonest sites. Onset is sudden, usually with loss of motor function down the opposite side of the body (*hemiplegia* or '*stroke*'), and, as bleeding is invariably progressive, death often ensues after a few days from raised intracranial pressure.

Subarachnoid haemorrhage, blood in the subarachnoid space, is usually due to a ruptured 'berry' aneurysm on one of the arteries in or around the circle of Willis (Chapter 12). Although the haemorrhage is maximal around the aneurysm, it mixes with CSF throughout the subarachnoid space, and is identifiable on lumbar puncture. Clinically, it presents as sudden, severe headache; features of meningeal irritation and raised intracranial pressure may also develop. Just over 50% of these patients die soon after their first bleed; some of the remainder are suitable for appropriate neurosurgery to prevent further haemorrhage. Occasionally, subarachnoid haemorrhage represents extension of intracerebral haemorrhage; this is invariably fatal.

Cerebral infarction

Cerebral infarction indicates inadequate cerebral blood flow, and is usually due to either arterial obstruction (e.g. by atheroma with or without superadded thrombus and thrombotic embolisation) or severe hypotension (e.g. anoxia during cardiac arrest). Any area may infarct, but that supplied by the middle cerebral artery is affected most commonly. Initially, cerebral infarcts are soft and swollen, due to colliquative ischaemic necrosis; they are usually pale, but may sometimes be haemorrhagic. Later, they become firmer and cystic ('*apoplectic cysts*') as replacement by gliosis occurs. Although clinical features depend on the site, most present with irreversible hemiplegia ('stroke'); prognosis is related to the underlying cause, but is usually fairly poor.

Head injuries

Head injuries are important causes of death and severe permanent disability, particularly in younger individuals; often road traffic accidents or falls are responsible. One or more of several lesions may be present.

Fractured skull

Fractured skull requires considerable force, and is usually, but not always, associated with significant brain damage; however, serious brain injury may occur without skull fractures. Most fractures increase the likelihood of subsequent acute meningitis.

Extradural haemorrhage

Extradural haemorrhage lies between the dura and skull; it is usually from a ruptured middle meningeal artery, and there is invariably an overlying skull fracture. The haemorrhage, which remains localised, gradually enlarges, producing raised intracranial pressure and, if untreated, death. Typically, there is a *lucid interval* between recovery from the initial trauma and deterioration from increased intracranial pressure.

Subdural haemorrhage

Subdural haemorrhage is from lacerated veins in the subdural space, and spreads over one or both hemispheres.

Acute subdural haemorrhage is common in severe head injuries and usually relatively unimportant. Occasionally, in less severe cases, it is large and behaves like an extradural haemorrhage.

Chronic subdural haemorrhage develops insidiously over several months, and often, particularly in the elderly, follows trivial injury without fracture. It slowly increases in size, and gradually produces raised intracranial pressure; if untreated, death ultimately occurs.

Brain damage

Contusions (i.e. bruises) and *lacerations*, produced by impact injury, are usually confined to the cortex. They are due to the brain moving within the cranial cavity, and thus are often found at both impact (*coup injuries*) and directly opposite (*contre coup injuries*) sites.

Diffuse damage is due to shearing and tearing of nerve fibres by rotational movement. It may be very severe, with deep irreversible coma, and yet macroscopic abnormalities are minimal; nerve fibre degeneration is seen histologically.

Intracerebral haemorrhage may be multiple, and usually reflects extensive damage with tearing of smaller blood vessels.

Oedema, secondary to most lesions just described, is common. If severe, it will contribute to raised intracranial pressure.

Hydrocephalus

Hydrocephalus is excess CSF, and may be primary or secondary.

Primary

Primary hydrocephalus is due to CSF pathway obstruction.

Congenital hydrocephalus usually follows either incomplete development of ventricles, foramina or aqueduct, or intra-uterine infections (e.g. toxoplasmosis and tuberculosis).

Acquired hydrocephalus develops in a previously normal brain, and is usually due to either some form of meningitis or tumours, especially of the brain stem.

Results vary with the degree of obstruction, and are influenced by surgical intervention (e.g. insertion of appropriate drains). Some ventricular system dilatation proximal to the obstruction will occur, and if it develops in infancy the cranium distends, with separation of skull sutures and gradual brain tissue destruction; if it develops after suture closure, skull enlargement cannot occur, but more rapid brain compression and destruction are produced. Continuing primary hydrocephalus causes raised intracranial pressure.

Secondary

Secondary hydrocephalus follows reduction in brain tissue volume—for example after cerebral infarction and in general paralysis of the insane. CSF pressure, and hence intracranial pressure, is not raised.

Demyelinating diseases

Demyelinating diseases show random myelin loss within the white matter with, at least initially, preservation of axis cylinders. Although usually chronic, it occasionally develops very acutely and is rapidly fatal (e.g. following viral infections or primary vaccinations); aetiology and pathogenesis are unknown, but abnormal immunological mechanisms are probably somehow responsible.

Disseminated (multiple) sclerosis shows multiple areas of demyelination (*plaques*) disseminated randomly throughout the brain and spinal cord. It usually presents in young adults, more commonly females, and, although a relapsing and remitting course is usual, the overall picture is often progressive deterioration. Plaques, which vary considerably in size, number and distribution, are usually grey in colour; later they become firm as axis cylinders are destroyed and replaced by gliosis. Clinically, neurological abnormalities reflect the patchy demyelination and include various motor, sensory and mental changes. Aetiology remains unknown; immunological mediation is probable, but as it is more common in temperate climates some additional environmental factor (e.g. viral) seems to be involved.

Degenerative diseases

Degenerative diseases are characterised by generalised or selective neurone loss.

Parkinson's disease is due to progressive loss in the substantia nigra, and produces muscular rigidity and tremor. The cause remains unknown.

Huntington's chorea, an autosomal dominant condition, is associated with generalised cortical neuronal loss; more extensive thalamic involvement causes the characteristic coarse involuntary choreiform movements.

Dementia represents severe generalised cortical atrophy and neuronal destruction producing progressive intellectual deterioration; it is usually due to ischaemia from severe cerebral artery atherosclerosis.

Raised intracranial pressure

Raised intracranial pressure is a serious complication of any expanding intracranial lesion and if unrelieved soon proves fatal.

Causes. These are numerous, and include haemorrhage (intracerebral, subarachnoid, subdural and extradural), massive infarction, cerebral oedema, hydrocephalus, brain abscesses, gummas and tumours.

Results. CSF pathways are compressed, gyri are flattened, sulci are narrowed and brain tissue is distorted and ultimately displaced (*brain shift*). Brain shift, easily identified by various radiological techniques, is away from the causative lesion, and produces herniation around the fixed septate projections of the dura mater.

Effects. These include persistent headache, vomiting, hypertension, bradycardia, cranial nerve palsies and impaired consciousness; later features are coma and, ultimately, death.

Treatment. This consists mainly of removing the cause surgically if possible, reducing cerebral oedema by drugs and, if necessary, draining CSF.

Tumours

Tumours may arise from neuroglia (gliomas), neurones (medulloblastoma), meninges (meningioma) and intracranial nerve roots, or may be metastatic. Primary brain tumours account for about 2% of all malignancies; metastatic tumours are much more frequent.

Gliomas

Gliomas are the commonest primary tumour. They infiltrate adjacent brain tissue (making complete surgical removal virtually impossible and thus producing a poor long term prognosis) but do not metastasise outside the nervous system. Several types, depending on the cell of origin, are described, and all show varying degrees of differentiation which correlate well with shorter term prognosis.

Astrocytomas comprise about 75% of gliomas. Most arise in adults, and are usually in cerebral hemispheres; a few develop in children, invariably in the cerebellum. Well-differentiated tumours are relatively slowly growing and are often either firmer than normal due to glial fibre production or cystic; poorly differentiated tumours are usually soft, with areas of haemorrhage and necrosis. Undifferentiated astrocytomas are fairly common, and are often called *glioblastoma multiforme*; they grow very rapidly, and soon prove fatal. Clinical and psychiatric symptoms are determined by tumour site, and often also include features of raised intracranial pressure. Prognosis is related to differentiation, and ranges from several years to a few months.

Medulloblastoma

Medulloblastomas are primitive nerve cell tumours. They invariably develop in childhood and usually arise in the cerebellum near the fourth ventricle. Local spread by infiltration soon produces hydrocephalus and raised intracranial pressure; meningeal seeding via CSF is common.

Meningioma

Meningiomas are the commonest meningeal tumours, and probably arise from arachnoid granulations. Although they may develop at any age and site, most present between 45 and 55 years, and the commonest locations are around the sagittal sinus, near the olfactory groove and the sphenoidal ridge. They are usually spherical, firm, slowly growing, well-demarcated tumours attached to meninges and indenting brain. Over 90% are benign and non-invasive; the remainder infiltrate adjacent bone and/or brain, but very few produce extracranial metastases. Symptoms relate to brain compression with neurological abnormalities and raised intracranial pressure. As most are benign, surgical removal is usually curative.

Schwannomas

Schwannomas (*neurilemmomas*) are peripheral nerve tumours probably derived from Schwann cells, but they may arise within the cranial cavity. Here, most develop on the acoustic nerve just inside the internal auditory meatus at the cerebello-pontine angle (*acoustic neuroma*); they grow slowly and compress adjacent brain, including the fourth ventricle, producing appropriate neurological disturbances such as cranial nerve palsies and raised intracranial pressure. Almost all are benign, but local recurrence following surgery is not uncommon.

Metastases

Metastatic tumours are very common, the most likely primary sites being bronchus and breast; multiple deposits are usual. It is not uncommon for patients to present with symptoms from cerebral metastases (e.g. neurological disturbances and raised intracranial pressure) before the primary tumour has become apparent clinically.

SPINAL CORD

Normal

The spinal cord occupies the upper two-thirds of the vertebral canal. It is continuous with the medulla oblongata, and is covered by the same protective membranes as the brain (i.e. dura mater, arachnoid and pia mater). It consists of central grey matter containing both descending motor and ascending sensory nerve fibre tracts and peripheral white matter, which gives rise to 31 pairs of spinal nerves; throughout, a supporting framework of neuroglia is present.

Inflammation

Some inflammation often accompanies most brain infections (e.g. acute bacterial, viral and tuberculous meningitis). Two particular lesions are considered here.

Poliomyelitis, infection by polio virus (usually type I), occurs both sporadically and in epidemics, but vaccination has reduced the disease considerably in more well-developed countries. The virus usually spreads via the faecal/oral route, and although its infectivity is high, most patients (typically children and young adults) are either asymptomatic or show only non-specific symptoms including pyrexia, malaise, sore throat and mild headache; few develop features of viral meningitis (see above) and even fewer, probably less than 1%, progress to paralysis. Such patients show asymmetrical and irregular degeneration and necrosis of spinal cord anterior (ventral) horn cells, with congestion, oedema and infiltration by lymphocytes, plasma cells, macrophages and occasional polymorphs; later, damaged nerve cells recover, but necrotic cells are replaced by gliosis. Extent and distribution of paralysis reflect severity and location of involvement; some improvement occurs as damaged nerve cells recover, but permanent flaccid paralysis indicates irreversible damage, and affected muscles show neurogenic atrophy (Chapter 23). Death is uncommon, but may occur if muscles of respiration are involved.

Tabes dorsalis is a late and relatively uncommon manifestation of tertiary syphilis (cf. general paralysis of the insane). It is slowly progressive degeneration and demyelination of posterior sensory columns with replacement by gliosis. It produces gradual loss of positional and pain sensation, mainly in lower limbs. Pathogenetic mechanisms are unknown.

Spinal cord compression

Spinal cord compression indicates local disruption and is sometimes referred to as a *transverse lesion.*

Causes. These are numerous and include vertebral column disorders (e.g. primary and secondary tumours, tuberculosis, fracture–dislocation, crush fractures and prolapsed intervertebral discs), extramedullary lesions (e.g. meningeal and nerve root tumours, metastases and extradural abscesses) and spinal cord lesions (e.g. gliomas, haemorrhage and infarction).

Results. The affected segment is swollen and distorted, with variable colliquative necrosis. In addition, motor tracts below and sensory tracts above the level of compression show degeneration and demyelination with associated motor and sensory dysfunction (e.g. paralysis and anaesthesia).

Syringomyelia

Syringomyelia is a rare condition, usually presenting in young adults, in which fluid-filled cavities and gliosis develop in the cervical cord. As the cavities enlarge and coalesce, local destruction produces both sensory abnormalities in upper limbs and face (mainly pain and temperature) and motor disturbances in the legs.

Subacute combined degeneration

Subacute combined degeneration of the cord is degeneration and demyelination of both motor and sensory tracts due to vitamin B_{12} deficiency (pernicious anaemia—Chapter 20); it is now virtually unknown where B_{12} therapy is available.

Motor neurone disease

Motor neurone disease is an uncommon condition of unknown aetiology showing progressive degeneration of anterior horn cells, cranial motor nuclei and spinal motor tracts; several different clinical types reflect different sites of maximal involvement. All present insidiously, mainly between 40 and 55 years, and are commoner in men. Progression is inevitable, with death after 2 to 5 years, usually from respiratory problems.

Tumours

Tumours are uncommon, and include astrocytoma, ependymoma, meningioma, Schwannoma and metastases (see brain tumours above); symptoms usually relate to local compression.

PERIPHERAL NERVES

Normal

They are ultimately branches of either the 12 pairs of cranial or the 31 pairs of spinal nerves, and contain both motor and sensory fibres.

Trauma

Trauma (transection, pressure or traction) is the commonest cause of damage. Initially, there is degeneration and demyelination of one or two proximal and all distal segments, followed by axis cylinder regeneration and Schwann cell proliferation within neurilemmal sheaths. If nerve fibre continuity is retained or restored surgically, axons grow down the corresponding sheaths at 2–3 mm per day until re-innervation is complete and normal function returns; if nerve fibre apposition is inadequate (e.g. interposition of other tissues) axonal sprouts, Schwann cells and fibroblasts proliferate to produce a *traumatic neuroma* at the site of injury, and functional recovery is poor or absent.

Peripheral neuropathy

Peripheral neuropathy indicates dysfunction; it is often still referred to as *neuritis*, although inflammation is rare.

Causes. These are numerous, and include vitamin deficiencies (especially B_1 and B_2), organic poisons (e.g. benzenes and carbon disulphide), metal poisons (e.g. lead and arsenic), drugs (e.g. isoniazid and sulphonamides), metabolic diseases (e.g. diabetes mellitus, porphyria, myxoedema and amyloidosis), infections (e.g. leprosy and tetanus), connective tissue diseases (Chapter 23), chronic alcoholism and carcinomatosis.

Results. All produce degeneration and demyelination, usually without any specific features to indicate the underlying cause.

Effects. Distribution is very variable, but often symmetrical and most marked in limbs. Affected nerves produce motor and/or sensory disturbances (e.g. weakness, pain and paraesthesia) in appropriate areas. If the cause is treated or removed, considerable axon regeneration with function restoration usually occurs; otherwise, there is gradual progression and extension.

Tumours

Tumours are probably derived from Schwann cells, and may be multiple. Depending largely on their collagen content, they are usually designated neurofibroma or Schwannoma; this distinction can be difficult, and is probably of limited value.

Neurofibromas present as diffuse, irregular swellings. They comprise spindle-shaped cells and collagen in which nerve fibres are embedded. Most are benign, but many recur after local excision; a few become malignant, usually after many years. When multiple, they may be associated with skin pigmentation (café au lait spots) and inherited as an autosomal dominant—*neurofibromatosis* or *von Recklinghausen's disease.*

Schwannomas (neurilemmomas) may be intracranial, intraspinal (see above) or peripheral. They are firm, encapsulated, discrete tumours, with a rather characteristic histological pattern of fibrocellular bundles containing regular rows of parallel spindle cells forming a 'palisade'; nerve bundles are usually stretched over the periphery. Local recurrence is common, but subsequent malignant change is rare.

EYE

Normal

The eye consists of two main chambers separated by the *lens* and *ciliary muscles.* The smaller *anterior chamber* contains *aqueous humour* and is limited anteriorly by the *cornea* with its covering of *conjunctiva*; just in front of the lens it contains the *iris.* The much larger *posterior chamber* contains *vitreous humour* and is limited posteriorly by the *retina* (containing specialised light-sensitive nerve cells), the vascular, pigmented *choroid* and the outer fibrous *sclera.*

Inflammation

Inflammation usually reflects infection, but may, particularly in the conjunctiva, represent reaction to foreign bodies, toxic agents or allergens; autoimmune reactions are occasionally responsible.

Viral conjunctivitis

Viral conjunctivitis is common, and usually due to adenoviruses or herpes virus (e.g. herpes zoster). Although the conjunctiva is primarily involved, extension into the cornea may occur, with ulceration, vascularisation, chronic inflammation and fibrosis; extensive scarring may lead to blindness.

Trachoma and inclusion conjunctivitis

These are caused by *Chlamydia* (Chapter 5). Extension from conjunctiva into superficial cornea with subsequent fibrosis and blindness is common.

Acute bacterial conjunctivitis

Acute bacterial conjunctivitis, due to pyogenic organisms (including gonococci), is now uncommon. Spread into cornea, iris and anterior chamber with pus formation usually occurs in untreated cases; then blindness in the affected eye is inevitable.

Keratitis

Keratitis, corneal inflammation, is often superficial. It usually represents direct spread from conjunctival infections, but is also a component of Sjögren's syndrome (Chapter 15). Healing by fibrosis produces visual impairment, and, if severe, blindness.

Interstitial keratitis, inflammation in deeper corneal layers, may follow superficial keratitis, but is often syphilitic and associated with syphilitic uveitis (see below). Dense, extensive fibrosis results.

Uveitis

Uveitis is inflammation of one or more components of the uveal tract—choroid (*choroiditis*), iris (*iritis*) and ciliary body (*cyclitis*).

Acute uveitis. This indicates pyogenic bacterial infection and abscess formation. It may follow conjunctivitis, penetrating wounds, pyaemia or septicaemia. There is considerable structural damage and blindness; retinal detachment is common.

Syphilis. Uveitis may occur in secondary or congenital syphilis, with visual disturbances or even, in severe cases, blindness.

Toxoplasmosis. Particularly if it is congenital (Chapter 5), toxoplasmosis may cause severe choroidal damage and blindness.

Autoimmune uveitis. Two forms exist. *Lens-induced uveitis* follows lens trauma, and is granulomatous inflammation due to both humoral and cell-mediated immune reactions. *Sympathetic*

ophthalmitis follows iris or ciliary body trauma, and produces cell-mediated granulomatous uveitis in the opposite eye, sometimes years after the initiating injury.

Glaucoma

Glaucoma, raised intra-ocular pressure following aqueous humour outflow obstruction, normally occurs in the acute angle between iris and cornea.

Types

Closed-angle glaucoma develops in individuals with unusually narrow irido-corneal angles when iris and lens come into contact and cause anterior bowing of the iris. Onset is usually fairly rapid.

Open-angle glaucoma develops insidiously. Normal anatomical relationships are preserved, but there is outflow tract obstruction (e.g. by collagen, chronic inflammation or tumour cells).

Results

Increased intra-ocular pressure impairs vascular perfusion and causes ischaemia of retinal nerve fibres; visual disturbances are produced, and without treatment (i.e. surgical drainage), blindness will result.

Cataract

Cataract is a lens opacity.

Causes. Most are related to ageing (*senile cataracts*), and represent acceleration of normal physiological sclerosis. Other causes include trauma and diabetes mellitus. Occasionally, they are congenital; these may be familial or due to intra-uterine rubella infection.

Results. Initially, visual disturbances are produced, but most progress gradually to blindness.

Tumours

Many primary tumours, both benign and malignant, are described; only two are relatively common. Metastases within the eye are unusual.

Malignant melanoma, derived from uveal tract

melanocytes, is the commonest intra-ocular tumour; over 80% arise in the choroid, usually posteriorly. Local growth often causes retinal detachment and secondary glaucoma; haematogenous spread produces metastases, particularly in the liver. Overall, prognosis is more favourable than for cutaneous malignant melanomas (Chapter 25), and over 50% are still alive at 5 years; however, at this site, it is well known for producing fatal, multiple hepatic metastases up to 20 years later, although reasons for this are unknown.

Retinoblastoma, derived from primitive retinal nerve cells, presents in infancy or early childhood, and is familial in 6% of cases; in almost 50% it is bilateral. Local growth soon produces retinal detachment and blindness, and there may be direct extension along the optic nerve into the brain; haematogenous metastases are uncommon and late. Prognosis is relatively good—over 80% survive.

DENTAL ASPECTS

Facial paralysis

Causes include a 'stroke' (cerebral infarction or intracerebral haemorrhage), facial nerve damage (by trauma, primary neoplasms or infiltrating parotid gland tumours) and Bell's palsy.

Bell's palsy is a facial nerve palsy presenting as unilateral facial paralysis. Aetiology is uncertain, but possibly inflammatory. A lop-sided appearance is produced when smiling, and saliva dribbles from the corner of the mouth on the affected side. When the patient attempts to close both eyes, the eyelids on the paralysed side fail to meet and the eyeball rotates upwards. Infection of the geniculate ganglion by the varicella–zoster (V–Z) virus produces similar paralysis (Ramsay–Hunt syndrome).

Neuralgias are recurrent bouts of intense, stabbing pain in sensory nerve pathway distributions. Examples include postherpetic, glossopharyngeal (affecting the pharynx and posterior tongue), sphenopalatine (affecting nose, eyes and temple) and trigeminal. Clearly, these and other causes of facial pain must be considered in the differential diagnosis of pulpitis.

Trigeminal neuralgia affects one or more branches of the trigeminal nerve to produce attacks of unilateral pain. Although each episode lasts only a few seconds, it is extremely painful, and patients may become depressed or even suicidal. Trigger zones which, when lightly touched, will initiate an attack may be present on the face or in the mouth. Patients readily identify such zones; their presence can lead to an avoidance of washing, shaving or eating.

25

Mucocutaneous diseases

Normal
Terminology
Inherited diseases
Bacterial diseases
Viral diseases
Fungal diseases

Bullous diseases
Drug-induced diseases
Hyperproliferative diseases
Connective tissue diseases
Lupus erythematosus
Progressive systemic sclerosis

Neoplasms
Benign epithelial
Malignant epithelial
Melanocytic neoplasms and naevi
Dermal

Normal

Skin is an extensive organ, and is continuous with the gastrointestinal, reproductive and urinary tracts. It is affected by disease as tissue in its own right, but also reflects disorders in other systems. Many skin diseases also involve mucous membranes; in this chapter, skin and oral mucosa are considered.

Skin and oral mucosa comprise epithelium (epidermis) and supporting connective tissues (dermis). The epithelium is stratified squamous, and consists of keratinocytes and non-keratinocytes. *Keratinocytes* are derived from the basal layer; they move upwards through spinous and granular layers and in skin are shed from the stratum corneum as *orthokeratinised* (i.e. anucleate) squames. Most oral mucosa (e.g. buccal and lip surfaces) lacks a stratum corneum; keratinisation, when present, is often *parakeratin*, where nuclear remnants are visible in the stratum corneum, and the stratum granulosum is absent or poorly formed. *Non-keratinocytes* include *melanocytes* (of neural crest origin, responsible for skin pigmentation), *Langerhans cells* (of bone marrow origin, important for immunological reactions in skin) and *Merkel cells* (also of neural crest origin, with a proprioceptive role and connections with dermal nerve fibres). In addition, specialised appendages are present in the dermis (e.g. hair follicles, sebaceous glands and sweat glands).

Terminology

The following are some common clinical and histological terms applied to skin:

Acanthosis. An increase in stratum spinosum cells, reflecting increased cell production in the basal layer. The epithelium is thickened, and may have prominent, wide epithelial rete ridges.

Hyperkeratosis. An increase in stratum corneum thickness. In the mouth, this produces a white appearance.

Atypia and *dysplasia*. These are discussed in Chapter 9.

Vesicle. A fluid-filled blister within or immediately below the epidermis (i.e. intra- or subepithelial); if greater than 5 mm in diameter, the term *bulla* is used.

Papule. A slightly raised surface lesion up to 1 cm in diameter.

Ulcer. A loss of continuity of any surface epithelium.

INHERITED DISEASES

Ectodermal dysplasia is an X-linked recessive condition producing abnormalities of skin, hair and teeth. Sweat and sebaceous glands are reduced or absent, so patients are sensitive to heat; hair is scanty, nail defects are common; deciduous and permanent dentitions may fail to develop.

Ichthyosis is a severe abnormality of keratinisation producing thick 'scales'. It may be an autosomal dominant, or a sex-linked recessive affecting males.

Ehlers–Danlos syndrome is characterised by collagen defects. The skin can be abnormally stretched, and bruising and bleeding occur due to increased capillary fragility. Joints can be easily dislocated, wound healing is impaired, and the mitral valve is 'floppy'. Dental abnormalities have been described, including poorly formed dentine, pulp stones and root formation defects.

BACTERIAL DISEASES

Acne vulgaris commonly affects adolescents. Hormonally induced increases in sebum production with blockage of pilosebaceous ducts lead to cystic dilatation of hair follicles of the face and upper body followed by bacterial colonisation and inflammation, with possible suppuration and scarring. The clinical hallmark is the comedone (blackhead), a hair follicle distended with keratin and sebum which ultimately ruptures onto the skin surface. Treatment is with antibiotics, such as tetracycline, but the disease regresses spontaneously with time.

Erysipelas is infection by *Streptococcus pyogenes*. The skin is swollen and red; the patient is quite unwell, and before antibiotics were available, death was common.

Impetigo is a contagious skin disease of young people caused by streptococci or staphylococci. Pustules and vesicles develop, often on the face.

Tuberculosis (*lupus vulgaris*) may be caused by atypical *Mycobacteria* as well as those responsible for classical tuberculosis.

VIRAL DISEASES

Herpes zoster (shingles) and *chickenpox* (varicella) are caused by the same virus. Initial infection is either subclinical or produces chickenpox (with skin rash, often on the torso, and fever) whilst reactivation causes shingles.

Herpes simplex can cause facial 'cold sores', herpetic whitlows of the fingers, and a severe form of eczema in infants.

Coxsackie viruses are responsible for *hand, foot and mouth disease*, presenting as oral ulcers, a skin rash often of the hands and feet, gastrointestinal upset and fever.

Measles is a contagious disease affecting children and characterised by fever, skin rash (usually of face, scalp and upper body) and transient, small whitish spots in the mouth (Koplik's spots); secondary bacterial infection, including bronchopneumonia, can occur.

Viral infections of skin and oral mucosa often produce vesicles which rupture to yield shallow ulcers. In the mouth in particular, these become secondarily infected by bacteria, inflamed and painful. Infected epithelial cells may contain inclusion bodies and may become multinucleate or degenerate. Viral warts are considered later as neoplasms.

FUNGAL DISEASES

Candidosis is mucosal infection (mouth and vagina) by *Candida albicans*; skin and finger nails are affected in *chronic mucocutaneous candidosis*. Such patients often have either immunological deficiencies, usually of T cells, or endocrine abnormalities.

Ringworm is infection by dermatophytes; scalp (tinea capitis) or feet (athlete's foot) are usually involved.

BULLOUS DISEASES

Bullous diseases produce large fluid- or blood-filled skin or mucosal blisters. An immunological basis is probable, as there are either circulating antibodies to epidermal components or local immunoglobulin deposits.

Pemphigus vulgaris usually affects people in late middle age. Although it can present in the mouth, many patients have both skin and oral involvement. Circulating antibodies in the blood (mainly IgG) are present to stratum spinosum cell membrane components, and antibody titre correlates with disease activity, being raised in active disease and low in remission. An underlying HLA basis might exist, as there is an increased incidence of HLA-A10 in affected patients. Antigen–antibody binding in the spinosum causes epidermal cells to produce proteinases which cause breakdown of cell contacts (acantholysis). Histologically, an intraepithelial, fluid-filled bulla is present, its floor lined by basal cells in contact with the dermis. The acantholytic spinosus cells are rounded and often lie free within the bullous cavity. The bullae are large and flaccid, and when they rupture give rise to ulcers which become secondarily infected. This and electrolyte loss used to cause death, but the disease responds to corticosteroids and healing occurs without scarring.

Benign mucous membrane pemphigoid affects conjunctivae and mucosae, particularly the mouth, of elderly patients; less than 50% have skin involvement. Histologically, epithelium and dermis separate at the basement membrane due to deposition of IgG and C3 in this zone; in only a few patients are circulating antibodies present. The bullae are tense, small and blood filled, and on rupturing, the ulcers become secondarily infected. Healing occurs with scarring, and, with conjunctival damage, blindness may eventually develop.

Bullous pemphigoid is seen in the elderly as large fluid-filled skin bullae; only one-third have oral involvement. IgG is always deposited at the basement membrane and circulating antibodies to a normal basal cell component are present in 70–80%. This antigen–antibody reaction activates complement, and C3 is also deposited. Polymorphs are attracted by activated complement components and release lysosomal enzymes responsible for the observed tissue damage and subepithelial bullae.

Dermatitis herpetiformis is an uncommon condition of middle age presenting as bouts of vesicular, bullous or erythematous skin papules; oral lesions are possible. Histologically, subepithelial bullae and numerous neutrophil and eosinophil polymorphs are present. The underlying cause may be sensitivity to dietary gluten (cf. coeliac disease, Chapter 16), as many patients also have small intestinal villous atrophy. Gluten combines with intestinal IgA to form immune complexes which are deposited at the dermo-epidermal junction, and the resulting damage is mediated by complement activation and subsequent polymorph chemotaxis. Over 90% of these patients express HLA-B8, suggesting a strong link with HLA-mediated disease.

DRUG-INDUCED DISEASES

Dermatitis is acute or chronic, and may be caused by numerous chemicals including antibiotics (e.g. penicillin and streptomycin), detergents, cosmetics, organic compounds (e.g. methyl methacrylate used in denture making) and toothpaste constituents. It presents as red, itchy, scaly, sometimes vesicular lesions at contact sites. Histological appearances vary from typical acute inflammation (with oedema, vascular dilatation, fibrin deposition and polymorph infiltration) producing epithelial vesiculation and parakeratosis in *acute dermatitis*, to chronic dermal inflammation with epithelial hyperkeratosis and acanthosis in *chronic dermatitis*. Agents causing dermatitis do so by damaging the skin (e.g. acids and alkalis) or by a type IV hypersensitivity reaction because either they are immunogenic by themselves or they act as haptens (Chapter 6) by combining with skin proteins to form antigenic complexes.

Erythema multiforme is a febrile illness affecting young adults, usually males. In 40 to 80% it is drug related (e.g. penicillin, sulphonamides, phenylbutazone and anti-epileptics), but may also follow viral infections (e.g. herpes simplex). Skin, mouth, eyes and genital mucosae can be involved. Skin lesions are circular and red, with concentric rings producing a 'target' or 'iris' appearance; oral lesions include swollen, bleeding and crusted lips with ulceration; conjunctival lesions may produce scarring and blindness. Histology shows vesiculobullous epithelial degeneration with inflammation in underlying connective tissues. Usually, it is self limiting, with healing after a few weeks; recurrences are possible, and severe cases (*Stevens–Johnson syndrome*) may prove fatal.

Lichen planus is included here as it can be caused by drugs (e.g. methyldopa, gold, phenolphthalein, antimalarials and antirheumatics); such cases are often referred to as 'lichenoid reactions', although clinically they are indistinguishable from non-drug-related cases. The latter are of unknown aetiology, but may be immunologically mediated. Skin lesions are itchy, red or purple papules, mainly on flexor surfaces of forearms and inner surfaces of legs; they may have whitish '*Wickham's striae*' running through them. Thirty to 70% of patients with skin lesions have oral involvement, but frequently the mouth is the only affected site, with, typically, a whitish network of hyperkeratosis (Wickham's striae) on cheeks and lips. It is usually symptomless, unless accompanied by inflammation or shallow ulceration (erosive lichen planus). Histology shows hyperkeratosis, para-

keratosis, a variably thickened stratum granulosum, pointed ('saw-tooth') rete ridges, oedema
and focal disruption of the basal layer ('liquefaction degeneration') with a 'band-like' infiltrate of
lymphocytes hugging the dermo-epidermal junction in which Civatte bodies (remnants of epithelial cells containing immunoglobulin deposits)
may be seen. Lichenoid reactions may also include
eosinophils.

HYPERPROLIFERATIVE DISEASES

Psoriasis is common, affecting up to 3% of the
population. It affects males and females equally,
and often begins in the second or third decades.
Clinically the skin bears discrete, slightly raised
plaques of keratinised squames. The nose, elbows
and knees are often affected; nails can be
involved, and some have joint problems (*psoriatic
arthritis*) resembling rheumatoid arthritis but
lacking rheumatoid factor. Oral lesions are very
uncommon. Histology reveals hyperkeratosis,
parakeratosis, acanthosis, elongated rete ridges
and dilated superficial dermal capillaries from
which polymorphs pass into the overlying epithelium to form superficial micro-abscesses. Psoriasis
is probably genetically determined, as many
patients express HLA-CW6, and those who
develop arthritis also express HLA-B27 (Chapter
6); in addition, there is depressed T cell and
increased monocyte activity. Pathogenesis is
unknown, but may involve production of antibodies to stratum corneum components with
injury helping to 'unmask' the antigens. The antibody–antigen complex binds and activates complement; activated C5 attracts polymorphs and
stimulates monocytes and macrophages to release
lymphokines which, in turn, induce the epithelial
proliferation that is the hallmark of the disease.
Treatment involves slowing down epithelial proliferation by cytotoxic drugs or PUVA therapy
(Chapter 11).

CONNECTIVE TISSUE DISEASES

Connective tissue diseases are considered collectively
and in more detail in Chapter 23.

Lupus erythematosus

Lupus erythematosus involving skin presents in two
forms.

Systemic lupus erythematosus (SLE) is a multi-
organ disease typically affecting young women.
Numerous immunological abnormalities are present,
including IgG and complement deposition in skin,
circulating antinuclear antibodies and LE cells.
The typical skin manifestation is a symmetrical
'butterfly' rash across the face and nose.

Discoid lupus erythematosus (DLE) is a localised,
mucocutaneous form with a better prognosis,
although a few cases eventually develop SLE. The
'butterfly' skin rash is present, and there may be
irregular oral mucosal ulcers. LE cells and circulating antibodies are much less common than in
SLE.

Progressive systemic sclerosis

Progressive systemic sclerosis is a multisystem
disease in which arterial narrowing produces
ischaemia and diffuse fibrosis. The skin becomes
stiff and the face adopts a characteristic, mask-
like, smiling appearance. Difficulties in opening
the mouth and chewing develop, and the oral
mucosa feels rigid and immobile. Radiologically,
many patients show widening of periodontal
ligaments.

NEOPLASMS

Primary neoplasms can develop from each cell
type within epithelium, hair follicles, sweat glands
or intradermal connective tissue.

Benign epithelial neoplasms

Basal cell papilloma (seborrhoeic keratosis) is a
very slowly growing warty nodule seen in old
people, especially on chest, back and forehead.
Microscopically, small, darkly staining epithelial
cells line cyst-like spaces filled with keratin.

Squamous cell papilloma is a warty growth
arising from either a slender stalk or a broader
base. Histologically, well-formed, stratified squamous epithelium covers a fronded core of fibrous

tissue. Growth is very slow, but trauma with secondary inflammation is common.

Viral warts can be single or multiple, and include the common *verruca vulgaris* (occurring mainly on the hands and sometimes in the mouth of children) and venereal warts (e.g. *condyloma accuminatum*). They are sessile or pedunculated, and often resemble squamous cell papillomas clinically and histologically. However, multiple lesions and inclusion bodies suggest a viral aetiology, and several associated human papilloma viruses have been described.

Keratoacanthoma (molluscum sebaceum) is an elevated, dome-shaped nodule with a central, keratin-filled crater. It is more frequent in old people, commonly occurs on the face and quickly enlarges over 2 or 3 months before undergoing spontaneous involution. Histologically, keratinous cysts and strands of regular squamous epithelium push downwards into the dermis over a broad front; characteristically, it elevates and undermines normal epithelium at its edges. Distinction from squamous cell carcinoma may be difficult both clinically and histologically. Treatment is by surgical removal, but recurrences occur, particularly on fingers and lips.

Malignant epithelial neoplasms

Basal cell carcinoma ('*rodent ulcer*') is the commonest malignant skin tumour. Typically, it is seen in the elderly, mainly on the face after prolonged exposure to ultraviolet radiation. It is a slowly growing ulcerated nodule with characteristic raised, rolled edges and a crusted centre. It is locally invasive, and if untreated may cause extensive destruction of facial bones and soft tissues, with extension into nasal passages, orbit and cranial cavity. Metastases are, for some unknown reason, extremely rare. Histologically, islands and strands (some cystic) of small, darkly-staining, basal-like cells of pilosebaceous origin invade the dermis; peripheral cells in the islands are often columnar in shape. Mitoses may be very numerous, but as there is considerable apoptotic cell death (Chapter 2) the lesion is only slowly growing. Patients with the autosomal dominant

Gorlin–Goltz syndrome (basal cell naevus syndrome) have multiple basal cell carcinomas, vertebral and rib anomalies, focal dura mater calcification and odontogenic keratocysts of the jaws.

Squamous cell carcinoma arises from such premalignant skin conditions as xeroderma pigmentosum and actinic keratosis (areas of collagen abnormality, epithelial atrophy and pigmentary changes in sun-exposed areas of outdoor workers) or develops de novo. Prognosis is reasonably good and considerably better than its oral counterpart (Chapter 15).

Melanocytic neoplasms and naevi

Hamartomatous abnormalities of melanocytes (or, more correctly, naevus cells) are common.

Naevi

In *intradermal naevi*, the commonest type, naevus cells form rounded masses in the dermis; the overlying epithelium is normal.

Junctional naevi show melanocyte aggregates within the epithelium at the dermo-epidermal junction.

Compound naevi show both intra-epidermal junctional and intradermal masses.

Most naevi are pigmented, and no treatment is required unless they enlarge, change colour or bleed; such lesions should be excised, as transformation to malignant melanoma, although very uncommon, is possible.

Malignant melanoma

Malignant melanoma arises either de novo (80%) or from a pre-existing naevus (20%). It may develop anywhere, although face, genitalia and feet are the commonest sites. Pigmentation is variable, but an enlarging, pigmented patch is often the presenting sign. Metastatic spread invariably takes place, particularly to lymph nodes, brain, liver, lungs and skin elsewhere. Histologically, several types exist, but it is the depth of dermal invasion which provides the greatest influence on prognosis. Thus, when the tumour is superficial (e.g. involvement of papillary dermis only) 5-year survival is 70–90%, but when it extends into subcutaneous fat the survival falls to 10–50%.

Dermal neoplasms

Dermal neoplasms are less common than epidermal tumours. They include fibroma, lipoma, angioma, neurofibroma and rarely, extranodal lymphoma. Occasionally, the dermis contains *metastatic carcinoma*, and this may represent the earliest manifestation of malignant disease elsewhere in the body.

Index

Abscess, 9
  brain, 129
  Brodie's, 119
  periapical, 11
Acantholysis, 139
Acanthosis, 138
Achalasia, 75
Achlorhydria, 76
Achondroplasia, 117
Acid phosphatase, 47
Acne vulgaris, 139
Acromegaly, 101
Actinomyces israelii, 18
Actinomycosis, 18
ADCC, 28, 31
Addison's disease, 29, 33, 103
Adenolymphoma, 73
Adenoma, 45
  monomorphic, 73
  pleomorphic salivary, 73
Adenovirus, 62, 135
Adhesions, 79
Adrenal gland, 102
Aetiology, 1
Aflatoxin, 43
Agenesis, 39
Agranulocytosis, 28, 108
AIDS, 28
Albers-Schonberg disease, 117
Aldosterone, 55
Alkaline phosphatase, 120
Alveolitis, cryptogenic fibrosing, 66
Ameloblastoma, 71
Amelogenesis imperfecta, 39
Amoebiasis, 21
Amyloid, 32, 65, 93, 116, 126
Anaemia, 47, 104
  aplastic, 106
  dyshaemopoietic, 105
  haemolytic, 29, 106
  hypoplastic, 106
  iron deficiency, 75, 105
  megaloblastic, 105
  pernicious, 105
Anaesthetic, general, 111
Anaphylaxis, 28
Aneurysm
  atheromatous, 53, 55
  berry, 55, 130

cardiac, 58
  dissecting, 55
  micro-, 55, 130
  mycotic, 55, 59
  syphilitic, 55
Angina, 38
Angioedema, hereditary, 27, 28
Angiofibroma, nasopharyngeal juvenile,
  62
Anisocytosis, 106
Ankylosis, 121
  bony, 123, 125
  fibrous, 123
Anthracosis, 33, 66
Antibody, 24
  cytotoxic, 28
Antibody-dependent cytotoxic cells, 25
Antibody response, 26
Antigen, 24
  Australia, 83
  carcinoembryonic, 47
Antinuclear factor, 126
Aorta, coarctation, 60
Aplasia, 39
  congenital thymic, 28
Apoptosis, 5, 49
Appendicitis, 77
Apud cells, 32, 45, 67, 102, 103
Apudoma, 45
Aqueous humour, 135
Arrhythmias, 58
Arteries, 52
Arteriolosclerosis, 54
Arteriosclerosis, 54
Arteritis, 53
Arthritis
  osteo-, 123, 127
  rheumatoid, 123
  tuberculous, 123
Arthus reaction, 29
Asbestos, 43, 66, 68
Aschoff nodules, 58
Aschoff-Rokitansky sinuses, 87
Ascites, 35, 80
Aspergillosis, 21, 65
Aspergillus
  flavus, 43
  fumigatus, 21, 130
Asthma, bronchial, 65

Astrocytoma, 133
Atheroma, 52
Atherosclerosis, 52, 57
Athlete's foot, 21, 139
Atrial septal defect, 59
Atrophy, 39
  brown, 34
  disuse, 39
  gastric, 76
  neurogenic, 125
  pressure, 39
  villous, 78, 140
Atypia, 41, 46, 138
Autograft, 24, 30
Autoimmune
  disease, 29
  reaction, 24
Autolysis, 4

Bacteraemia, 16
Bell's palsy, 137
Bence-Jones protein, 109
Bergonie and Tribondeau, law of, 48
Bilharziasis, 97, 98
Bilirubin, 34, 86
Bladder, 97
Bleeding time, 110
Blood clot, 36
Bone, woven, 13
Bone marrow ablation, 49
Brain
  damage, 131
  shift, 132
Bronchiectasis, 65
Bronchitis, chronic, 65
Bronchopneumonia, 63
Brucellosis, 116
Bulla, 66, 138
Bullous diseases, 139
Burns, 5
Bursa of Fabricius, 24

Cachexia, 39, 47
Caisson disease, 38
Calcification
  dystrophic, 32, 52, 58
  heterotopic, 32
  metastatic, 33, 102
Calculus, 87, 94, 102

Callus, 13, 118
Candida albicans, 21, 22, 71, 75, 130, 139
Candidosis, 21, 22, 28, 31, 139
  acute atrophic, 23
  acute pseudomembranous, 23
  chronic atrophic, 23
  chronic hyperplastic, 70
  chronic mucocutaneous, 139
Capillaries, 56
Carcinogenesis, 42
Carcinogens, 43
Carcinoma, 45
  adenoid cystic, 74
  basal cell, 142
  bronchogenic, 66
  in situ, 46, 70
  in pleomorphic adenoma, 74
  nasopharyngeal, 44, 66
  oat cell, 67
  oral, 71
  scar, 67
  verrucous, 71
Carcinomatosis, 46
  peritonei, 80
Cardiac
  failure, 58, 60
  tamponade, 58, 60
Cardiospasm, 75
Cat scratch disease, 114
Cataract, 136
Cell damage, 4
Cementoma, 72
Cerebrovascular
  accident, 130
  disease, 130
Chancre, 19
Cheilitis, angular, 23, 105
Chemotaxis, 8, 27
Cherubism, 117
Chickenpox, 139
Chlamydia, 20, 98, 136
Cholangiocarcinoma, 86
Cholecystitis, 86
Cholelithiasis, 87
Chondrocalcinosis, 124
Chondrosarcoma, 121
Choroiditis, 136
Christmas disease, 111
Chromosome, 'Philadelphia', 109
Chronic inflammation, 9
Cirrhosis, 36, 84
Civatte bodies, 141
Claudication, intermittent, 38
Cloacae, 119
Clostridium welchii, 5, 107, 124
Clotting, 36, 110
  time, 110
Cloudy swelling, 4
Coagulation, blood, 36, 110
Coarctation of the aorta, 60
Cobblestone appearance, 78, 81
Coeliac disease, 29, 70, 78, 81, 140
Collagen disease, 125
Commensal organisms, 15

Complement, 8, 27, 28
Condyloma accuminatum, 142
Condylomata lata, 19
Congestion, 35
  venous, 82
Conjunctivitis, 135
Connective tissue diseases, 125, 141
Contra suppressor T cells, 25
Cor pulmonale, 60
Coronary artery disease, 57
Coxa vara, 120
Coxiella burnetii, 20
Crescents, 93
Cretinism, 101
Crohn's disease, 70, 78, 81
Cryosurgery, 6
Cryptococcosis, 21, 65
Cryptococcus neoformans, 21, 130
Cyanosis, 60
Cyclitis, 136
Cyst
  apoplectic, 131
  branchial, 41
  dentigerous, 41
  dermoid, 41
  developmental, 41
  fissural, 41
  globulomaxillary, 41
  mucous extravasation, 72
  mucous retention, 72
  thyroglossal, 41
Cystic hygroma, 41
Cystitis, 97
Cytokeratin, 47
Cytomegalovirus, 72, 96
Cytotoxic T cells, 25

Dane particle, 83
Degeneration
  hyaline, 4
  hydropic, 4
Dementia, 132
Demyelinating disease, 132
Dental caries, 31, 69
  plaque, 69
Dentinoma, 72
Dermatitis, 140
  contact, 29
  herpetiformis, 29, 140
Dermatomyositis, 124, 126
Desmin, 47
Diabetes mellitus, 16, 89, 93
Diffferentiation of neoplasms, 44
Diffuse alveolar damage, 66
Diphyllobothrium latum, 105
Disseminated
  intravascular coagulation, 36, 111
  (multiple) sclerosis, 132
Diverticular disease, 78
Diverticulitis, 79
Diverticulosis, 79
DNA repair, 44
D₀, 48
Duchenne's muscular dystrophy, 125
Ductus arteriosus, 60

Dwarfism, 100
Dysphagia, 75
Dysplasia, 41, 138
  ectodermal, 138
  fibrous, 117, 121

Eburnation, 124
ECHO, 59
Effusion
  pericardial, 35, 60
  pleural, 35, 67
Elephantiasis, 36
Embolism, 37, 53
Embolus
  air, 37
  amniotic fluid, 38
  fat, 37
  paradoxical, 37, 59
  pulmonary, 37, 63
  saddle, 37
  systemic, 37, 53
  venous, 37
Emphysema, 65
Empyema (pyothorax), 64, 67
  of the gallbladder, 87
Encephalitis, 128
Enchondroma, 121
Endarteritis obliterans, 19, 50, 130
Endocarditis
  infective, 59
  non-bacterial thrombotic, 59
  rheumatic, 58
  subacute bacterial, 59
Endotoxins, 15
Entamoeba histolytica, 77
Eosinophilia, 108
Eosinophilic granuloma of bone, 121
Epithelioid cells, 17
Epulis
  gingival, 40
  pregnancy, 56
Erysipelas, 139
Erythema multiforme, 140
Erythroplakia, 70
Escherichia coli, 15, 36, 59, 91, 128
Exotoxin, 15, 16
Exudate, 35, 67
Eye, 135

Facial paralysis, 137
Fallot's tetralogy, 60
Fatty change, 4, 84
Fatty streaks, 52
Fc receptors, 25
Fibrillation, 124
Fibrin, 8
Fibrinolysis, 37, 110
Fibroblast stimulating factor, 27
Fibroblasts, 12
Fibrocystic disease (mucoviscidosis), 88
Fibroma, ossifying, 118, 121
Fibrosis, 9, 10
  progressive massive, 66
  submucous, 70
Filaments, intermediate, 47

Filariasis, 36, 56
Finger clubbing, 47
Floppy mitral valve, 58
Foetor hepaticus, 85
Fracture
  bone, 13
  comminuted, 118
  compound, 118
  greenstick, 118
  pathological, 118
  simple, 118
  spontaneous, 118
Fractured skull, 131
Frostbite, 6
Fungi, 21

Gallbladder, 86
Gallstones, 87
Ganglioneuroma, 103
Gangrene, 5
  gas, 5, 124
Gastritis, 76
  atrophic, 76
  autoimmune, 76, 105
Gastroenteritis, 76
Gaucher's disease, 4
General paralysis of the insane, 130
Genetic disease, 2
Ghon focus, 17, 64
Giant cells, 10
Gigantism, 100
Gingivitis, 31
Glandular fever, 114
Glaucoma, 136
Glioblastoma multiforme, 133
Glioma, 132
Gliosis, 13
Glomerulonephritis, 92, 126
Glossitis, median rhomboid, 23
Glucose-6-phosphate dehydrogenase,
  106
Glutamic oxalo-acetic transaminase, 58
Gluten, 78, 140
Glycogen storage disease, 4
Goitre, 101
Gonococcus, 98, 136
Gonorrhoea, 98
Gout, 33, 123, 124
Graft
  reaction, 30
  versus host disease, 30
Grafts
  allogeneic, 24
  syngeneic, 24
Granulation tissue, 9, 12, 33, 10, 64,
  78
Granuloma, 114
  apical, 11
  pyogenic, 56
Granuloma of bone, eosinophilic, 121
Graves' disease, 101
Gumma, 19, 119, 130
Gynaecomastia, 85

Haemangioendothelioma, 86

Haemangioma
  capillary, 40
  cavernous, 40
Haematocrit, 104
Haematoma, 36, 110
Haematuria, 93, 98
Haemochromatosis, 34, 85
Haemoglobinopathies, 106
Haemolytic disease of the newborn,
  34, 107
Haemopericardium, 36, 58, 60
Haemoperitoneum, 36
Haemophilia, 111
haemophilus influenzae, 59, 64
Haemorrhage, 36
  extradural, 131
  intracerebral, 130
  subarachnoid, 130
  subdural, 131
Haemorrhagic states, 110
Haemosiderin, 33
Haemosiderosis, 33
Haemothorax, 36, 67
Hamartoma, 40, 80
Hand, foot and mouth disease, 139
Hand-Schüller-Christian disease, 122
Hapten, 24, 26
Hashimoto's disease, 101
Head injury, 131
Healing, 12
Heart, 57
  disease, congenital, 59
  failure, 60
  failure cells, 35, 63
Heat, 6
Heberden's nodes, 124
Helper T cells, 25
Hemiplegia, 130, 131
Henoch-Schönlein purpura, 111
Hepatitis
  acute, 83
  alcoholic, 84
  B virus, 16, 99
  infectious, 83
  lupoid, 84
  non-A non-B, 83
  serum, 83, 90
Hepatization
  grey, 64
  red, 64
Hepatoma, 85
Hernia, 79
  hiatus, 76
Herpes
  labialis, 22
  simplex, 22, 31, 44, 83, 129, 139,
    140
  virus, 16
  zoster, 22, 135, 139
Herpetic
  gingivostomatitis, 22
  whitlow, 22
Heterograft, 24, 30
Heterotopia, 41
Histamine, 8

Histiocytosis X, 121
Histogenesis of neoplasms, 44
Histoplasma capsulatum, 21
Histoplasmosis, 21, 65
HLA system, 29, 70, 123, 139, 140,
  141
Hodgkin's disease, 114
Homograft, 24, 30
Huntington's chorea, 132
Hutchinson's incisor, 20
Hydrocephalus, 129, 131
Hydronephrosis, 94
Hydrophobia, 130
Hydrops fetalis, 107
Hydrothorax, 35
Hydroureter, 97
Hygroma, cystic, 41
Hyperaemia, 8, 35
Hypercalcaemia, 47, 102, 114
Hyperkeratosis, 138
Hyperlipidaemia, 53
Hypernephroma, 96
Hyperparathyroidism, 94, 95, 102
Hyperplasia
  denture irritation, 40
  epanutin, 40
  prostatic, 94, 98
  pseudo-epitheliomatous, 40
  reactive, 9
Hypersensitivity
  delayed, 27, 29
  reaction, 24, 28
Hypertension
  benign, 54, 94
  malignant, 54, 94, 107
  portal, 75, 85, 116
  pulmonary, 63
  secondary, 92, 93, 94
  systemic, 53, 54
Hyperthyroidism, 101
Hypertrophy, 39, 40
Hyphae, 21
Hypochlorhydria, 76
Hypogammaglobulinaemia
  infantile, 28
  X-linked, 28
Hypoglycaemia, 47, 89
Hypoparathyroidism, 102
Hypoplasia, 39
Hypothermia, 6, 88

Iatrogenic, 3
Ichthyosis, 138
Ileus, paralytic, 79
Immune
  system, 24
  complex, 29, 92, 125, 126,
    140
Immunity, 24, 26
Immunodeficiency, 27
  T cell, 116
Immunoglobulin, 24
Impetigo, 139
Incompetence, valvular, 58
Induration, brown, 63

Infarct, 38
  septic, 38
Infarction, 5, 38, 53, 82, 130
  cerebral, 130
  myocardial, 57
Infections, 15
  opportunistic, 28
Infectious mononucleosis, 114, 116
Infiltrations, 4
Inflammation, 7, 9
Initiation, tumour, 42
Interferon, 27
Interleukin, 27
Intestines, 77
Intracranial pressure, 132
Intrinsic factor, 105
Intussusception, 79
Involucrum, 119
Iritis, 136
Ischaemia, 38, 52
Ischaemic heart disease, 57

Jaundice 85, 86
Joint temporomandibular, 127
Joints, 123

Karyolysis, 4
Karyorrhexis, 4
Keratitis, 136
Keratoacanthoma, 142
Keratosis,
  actinic, 142
  oral, 99
  seborrhoeic, 141
Kernicterus, 107
Kidneys, 91
Killer cells, 25
Kimmelstiel-Wilson nodules, 93
Kinins, 8, 27
Klebsiella, 64
Koilonychia, 105
Koplik's spots, 139
Kveim test, 114

Lactic dehydrogenase, 58
Langerhans cells, 29, 30, 138
Langhans giant cells, 17
Larynx, 62
LE cells, 126
Leishmaniasis, 21
Leprosy, 18
Letterer-Siwe disease, 122
Leucocytes, 107
Leucocytosis, 107
Leucopaenia, 107
Leukaemia, 109
Leukoderma (vitiligo), 33
Leukoplakia, 23, 70
  candidal, 23
Lichen planus, 140
Lichenoid reaction, 140
Linear energy transfer, 48
Lingual thyroid, 41
Lipofuscin, 34

Liver, 82
  failure, 85
  palms, 85
Lobar pneumonia, 64
Loose bodies, 124
Lung collapse, 63
Lungs, 63
Lupus
  erythematosus, 141
  erythematosus, discoid, 141
  erythematosus, systemic, 126, 141
  vulgaris, 139
Lymphadenitis, 9, 113
Lymphadenopathy, 56, 113
Lymphangioma, 40
Lymphangitis, 9, 56
Lymphatics, 56
Lymph nodes, 113
Lymphocyte mitogenic factor, 27
Lymphocytes
  B, 9, 24
  T, 9, 24
Lymphocytosis, 108
Lymphoedema, 56
Lymphoepithelioma, 62
Lymphogranuloma inguinale, 20
Lymphokines, 24, 26
Lymphoma, 45, 114, 122
  Hodgkin's, 114
  non-Hodgkin's, 115
  Burkitt, 115
Lymphopaenia, 108
Lymphotoxin, 27

Macroglossia, 32
Macrophage, 8, 9, 10, 12, 25
Macrophage inhibition factor, 27
Malabsorption, 78, 105
Malaria, 21, 107, 116
Mean corpuscular
  volume, 104
  haemoglobin, 104
Measles, 114, 139
Meckel's diverticulum, 76, 78
Medulloblastoma, 133
Melanin, 33
Melanoma, malignant, 71, 136, 142
Melanosis coli, 33
Meningioma, 133
Meningitis
  bacterial, 128
  tuberculous, 129
  viral, 129
Merkel cells, 138
Mesothelioma, 43, 66, 68
Metaplasia, 41
  mucous, 41
  osseous, 41
  squamous, 41, 65, 67
Metastasis, 44, 67, 68, 86, 96, 114, 122, 133
Microaneurysm, 55, 130
Minimal change disease, 93
Minimal erythema dose, 50
Molluscum sebaceum, 142

Monocytes, 8
Monocytosis, 108
Mosaic appearance, 120
Motor neurone disease, 134
Mucocoele, 72
Mucoviscidosis, 88
Multinucleated giant cells, 9
Multiple myeloma, 32, 108
Mumps, 72, 88, 129
Muscular dystrophy, 125
Myasthenia gravis, 116, 125
Mycobacterium
  bovis, 113
  leprae, 18
  tuberculosis, 17, 64, 77
Mycoplasma pneumoniae, 21
Myelofibrosis, 106, 108
Myeloma, multiple, 25, 32, 108
Myocarditis
  non-inefective, 59
  toxic, 59
  viral, 58
Myocytes, 124
Myofibroblasts, 13
Myopathies, 47
Myositis, 124
  ossificans, 125
Myxoedema, 101

Naevus
  compound, 142
  intradermal, 142
  junctional, 142
  spider, 85
Nasopharyngeal juvenile angiofibroma, 62
Natural killer cells, 25
Necrosis
  avascular, 118
  caseous, 5, 17
  coagulative, 5, 19, 38, 44, 58
  colliquative, 5, 38, 130, 134
  fat, 5, 88
  fibrinoid, 5, 54, 125, 126
  piecemeal, 84
  suppurative, 5
  renal tubular, 36, 95
Negri bodies, 129
Neisseria
  gonorrhoeae, 98, 136
  meningitidis, 128
Neoplasia, 41
Neoplasms, 42
  odontogenic, 71
Nephroblastoma (Wilms' tumour), 96
Neuralgia, 137
  trigeminal, 137
Neurilemmoma, 133, 135
Neuritis, 135
Neuroblastoma, 103
Neurofibroma, 135
Neurofibromatosis, 135
Neuroma
  acoustic, 133
  traumatic, 135

Neuropathy, peripheral, 106, 135
Neurotrophic joint disease, 124
Neutropaenia, cyclical, 28, 108
Nitrosamines, 43
Nose, 62
Nutmeg liver, 35, 60, 82

Obstruction
  intestinal, 79
  oesophageal, 75
Odontomes, 41
Oedema, 35, 63, 131
Oesophagitis, 75, 76
Oesophagus, 75
Ollier's disease, 121
Oncogenes, 43
Oncornavirus, 43
Organisation, 9, 10, 12, 37
Ornithosis, 20
Ossification
  endochondral, 117
  metaplastic, 41
Osteitis fibrosa cystica, 102
Osteoarthritis, 123, 127
Osteoarthropathy, hypertrophic, 47
Osteoarthrosis, 123
Osteoblastoma, benign, 121
Osteocartilaginous exostosis, 121
Osteochondritis, 119
Osteochondroma, 121
Osteoclast-activating factor, 27
Osteoclastoma, 121
Osteogenesis imperfecta, 117
Osteolysis, 122
Osteoma, osteoid, 121
Osteomalacia, 120
Osteomyelitis, 16, 50, 119
Osteopetrosis, 117
Osteophytes, 124
Osteoporosis, 120
  circumscripta, 120
Osteoradionecrosis, 50, 51, 119
Osteosarcoma, 121
Osteosclerosis, 122

Packed cell volume, 104
Paget's disease of bone, 14, 120
Pancarditis, 58
Pancreas, 88
Pancreatitis, 88
Pancytopaenia, 106, 108
Pannus, 125
Papilloma, 45, 63
  basal cell, 141
  squamous cell, 141
Papule, 138
Paramyxovirus, 72
Parathyroids, 102
Parkinson's disease, 132
Pathogenesis, 1
Paul-Bunnell test, 114
Pel-Ebstein fever, 114
Pemphigoid
  benign mucous membrane, 140
  bullous, 140

Pemphigus vulgaris, 139
Pericarditis
  constrictive, 61
  fibrinous, 60
  rheumatic, 58
  suppurative, 60
  tuberculous, 61
Pericardium, 60
Periodontal disease, 31
Periodontitis, 31, 69
Periostitis, 119
Peripheral nerve, 134
Peritoneum, 80
Peritonitis, 77, 78, 80
Petechiae, 36, 110
Phaeochromocytoma, 103
Phagocytosis, 8
Phlebothrombosis, 37, 55
Pigeon chest, 120
Pigmentation, 33
Pituitary, 100
Plaque
  atheromatous, 52
  dental, 69
  fibrous pleural, 66
Plasma cells, 9
Plasmacytoma, 109
Plasmodium, 21
Pleomorphism, 44
Pleura, 67
Pleurisy, 67
Pneumococcus, 64
Pneumoconiosis, 66
Pneumocystis carinii pneumonia, 28
Pneumonia, 63
Pneumothorax, 67
Poikilocytosis, 106
Poison theory, 48
Polarity, 44
Poliomyelitis, 133
Polyarteritis nodosa, 53, 127
Polycystic disease, 91
Polycythaemia, 108
Polymorphs, 8, 9
Polymyositis, 124, 127
Polyp
  adenomatous, 79
  fibroepithelial, 40
  nasal, 62
Polyposis coli, 79
Porphyria, 34
Precarcinogens, 43
Premalignancy, 45, 70
Primary complex, 17, 64
Prognathism, 101
Promotion, tumour, 42
Proteinuria, 93
Proteus, 36
Protozoa, 21
Pseudomonas, 36
Psoriasis, 29, 141
Pulpitis, 10, 69
Purpura, 110
  thrombocytopaenic, 110
Puva therapy, 50, 141

Pyaemia, 16
Pyelonephritis, 91, 97
Pyknosis, 4

Q fever, 20

Rabies, 129
Rad, 48
Radiation
  ionising, 43, 48
  non-ionising, 50
  ultraviolet, 43, 50
Radiosensitisers, 51
Radiotherapy, 50
Raised intracranial pressure, 132
Ranula, 72
Raynaud's phenomenon, 126
Receptors, Fc, 25
Reed-Sternberg cell, 115
Regeneration, 9, 12
Rejection, graft, 30, 95
Relative biological efficiency, 48
Renal failure, 95
Renin-angiotensin system, 55
Reproductive death, 49
Resolution, 9, 12
Reticulocyte, 106
Retinoblastoma, 137
Reverse transcriptase, 43
Rheumatic
  diseases, 125
  fever, 29, 58
Rheumatoid
  factor, 30, 125
  nodules, 126
Rhinitis, 62
Rickets, 120
  hypophosphataemic vitamin D
    resistant, 120
Rickettsiae 20
Rickety rosary 120
Ringworm 139
Rubella 83

Sabre tibia, 120
Salivary gland, 72
Salmonella typhi, 77
Saprophyte, 15
Sarcoidosis, 114
Sarcoma, 45
  Kaposi's, 28
  osteogenic, 121
  synovial, 124
Schistosoma haematobium, 97
Schistosomiasis, 97, 98
Schwannoma, 133, 135
Scleroderma, 126
Sclerosis Monckeberg's medial, 53
  progressive systemic, 126, 141
Selective immunoglobulin deficiency,
  28
Septicaemia, 16, 116, 119
Sequestrum, 119
Serum markers of malignancy, 47
Serum sickness, 29

Shigella, 77
Shingles, 22, 139
Shock
  cardiogenic, 36
  hypovolaemic, 36
  liver, 82
  septic, 36
Sialadenitis, 72
Sickle cell disease, 107
Siderosis, 33
Silicosis, 66
Simmond's disease, 100
Singer's nodes, 63
Sinusitis, 62
Skeletal muscle, 124
Skin reactive factor, 27
Socket, dry, 14, 119
Spherocytosis, 106
Spinal cord, 133
  compression, 134
  degeneration of, 106, 134
Spirochaetes, 19
Spleen, 116
Splenomegaly, 85, 116
Spondylitis, ankylosing, 29, 123
Spotted fever, 129
Spread of malignant neoplasms, 46
Staphylococcus, 64
  aureus, 23, 59, 72
Starling's hypothesis, 8
Status asthmaticus, 65
Stem cell, 42
Stenosis
  calcific aortic, 58
  rheumatic valvular, 58
Still's disease, 125
Stomach, 76
Stomatitis nicotina, 72
Streptococcus, 64, 72
  β haemolytic, 58
  faecalis, 59
  mutans, 31
  pneumoniae, 128
  pyogenes, 139
  viridans, 15, 59
Sublethal damage, 49
Sulphur granules, 18
Suppressor T cells, 25
Suppuration, 9
Syndrome
  adrenogenital, 103
  Albright's, 117
  basal cell naevus, 142
  Caplan's, 126
  cerebral, 49
  Conn's, 103
  Cushing's, 16, 47, 101, 103
  Di George's, 28
  Ehlers-Danlos, 138
  fat embolism, 37
  Frohlich's, 100
  Gardner's, 79, 81
  gastrointestinal, 49
  Goodpasture's, 92
  Gorlin-Goltz, 142

Lorain-Levi's, 100
Maffucci's, 121
multiple endocrine neoplasia, 103
nephrotic, 36, 93
pain dysfunction, 127
Paterson-Kelly, 75, 76, 105
Peutz Jeghers, 33, 80, 81
Plummer Vinson, 75
Ramsay-Hunt, 137
Reiter's, 98, 99
Sheehan's, 100
Sjögren's, 72, 126, 136
Stevens-Johnson, 140
Waterhouse-Friderichsen, 129
Synovioma, 124
Synovitis, pigmented villonodular, 124
Syphilis, 19, 55, 114, 119, 130, 134, 136
Syringomyelia, 134

Tabes dorsalis, 133
Target theory, 48
Tattoo, amalgam, 33
Telangiectasia, hereditary
  haemorrhagic, 40, 111
Teratoma, 45
Tetany, 102
Thalassaemia, 107
Thrombocythaemia, 108, 111
Thrombocytopathia, 111
Thrombophlebitis, 55
  migrans, 47, 55
Thrombosis, 36, 52, 54
Thrombus, mural, 37
Thrush, 23
Thymoma, 116, 125
Thymus, 116
Thyroid, 101
Thyroiditis, autoimmune, 101
Thyrotoxicosis, 29, 30, 101
Tinea capitis, 139
Tolerance, 24
Tophi, 33, 123
Toxoid, 26
Toxoplasma gondii, 22
Toxoplasmosis, 22, 28, 114, 130, 131, 136
Trachoma, 20, 136
Transcoelomic spread of neoplasms, 46
Transplantation, 95
Transudate, 35, 67
Trench-foot, 6
Treponema pallidum, 19
Trichinella spiralis, 32
Trypanosomiasis, 21
Tuberculosis, 17, 61, 64, 66, 92, 113, 116, 119, 123, 129, 131, 134, 139
  miliary, 17, 64
Tumour, 42
  acinic cell, 74
  brain, 132
  brown, 102
  carcinoid, 79
  Ewing's, 121
  giant cell, 121

islet cell, 89
mucoepidermoid, 74
Sternberg, 116
transitional cell, 97
Warthin's, 73
Wilms', 96
Typhoid, 116
Typhus, 20

Ulcer, 138, 13
  rodent, 142
  snail-track, 19
Ulceration
  aphthous, 13, 69, 81
  herpetiform, 70
  oral, 13
  peptic, 76
  recurrent oral, 69, 105, 108
Ulcerative colitis, 70, 78, 81
Union
  delayed, 118
  primary, 12
  secondary, 13
Ureters, 97
Urethra, 98
Urethritis, non-specific, 98
Uveitis, 136

Varicella, 139
Varicella-zoster virus, 137
Varices, oesophageal, 75, 85
Varicose veins, 55
Vascular hamartoma, 40
Vasculitis, 29, 53
Vasculosis, plasmatic, 5
Veins, varicose, 55
Ventricular
  failure, 63
  septal defect, 60
Verruca vulgaris, 142
Vesicle, 138
Vibrio cholerae, 77
Vimentin, 47
Virilism, 103
Virulence, 15
Virus, 18, 43
  Coxsackie, 59, 139
  DNA tumour, 43
  Epstein-Barr, 44, 83, 114
  herpes simplex, 22, 31, 44, 83, 129, 139, 140
  influenza, 59
  RNA tumour, 43
  slow, 18
  varicella-zoster, 137
Vitamin D deficiency, 120
Vitreous humour, 135
Volvulus, 79
Von Willebrand's disease, 111
Von Recklinghausen's disease, 135

Waldenstrom's macroglobulinaemia, 109
Wart, viral, 142
Warthin-Finkeldy giant cell, 114

Wasserman reaction, 20
Wegener's granulomatosis, 54
White blood cells, 107
Wickham's striae, 140
Wilson's disease, 85

Xenograft, 24
Xeroderma pigmentosum, 142
Xerostomia, 51

Yeast, 21

Ziehl-Neelsen stain, 18